Trade Union Strategies against Healthcare Marketization

Marketization in the healthcare sector affects the quality and delivery of care, as well as healthcare workers' working conditions. Based on a comparison of England and Germany, along with an in-depth case study looking at New York, USA, this volume examines how trade unions respond to marketization processes and the determinants of successful strategies.

The author draws on a rich empirical study to develop a theoretical framework that accounts for sector-specific opportunity structures stemming from marketization processes and on the relevant unions' local-level leeway that opens if they build up and mobilize the available resources and capacities. The book identifies determinants of successful trade union strategies, explains the puzzling observation of similar strategic choices across different systems, and draws conclusions for prospects of trade unionism in the marketized healthcare sector. This book emphasizes the transformative effect of marketization on healthcare and the opportunities this change creates for unions, while giving special attention to the local-level conditions of trade unionism in the analysis of conflicts evolving around marketization in the hospital sector.

It is of interest to academics and practitioners working in healthcare management, human resource management, and employment relations.

Jennie Auffenberg is a Policy Advisor at the Bremen Chamber of Labour, Germany.

Routledge Key Themes in Health and Society

https://www.routledge.com/Routledge-Key-Themes-in-Health-and-Society/
book-series/RKTHS

Trade Union Strategies against Healthcare Marketization

Opportunity Structures and Local-Level Determinants

Jennie Auffenberg

Routledge
Taylor & Francis Group

LONDON AND NEW YORK

First published 2022
by Routledge
2 Park Square, Milton Park, Abingdon, Oxon OX14 4RN

and by Routledge
605 Third Avenue, New York, NY 10158

Routledge is an imprint of the Taylor & Francis Group, an informa business

© 2022 Jennie Auffenberg

British Library Cataloguing-in-Publication Data
A catalogue record for this book is available from the British Library

Library of Congress Cataloging-in-Publication Data
A catalog record has been requested for this book

ISBN: 978-0-367-47276-4 (hbk)
ISBN: 978-1-032-04330-2 (pbk)
ISBN: 978-1-003-03458-2 (ebk)

Typeset in Goudy
by KnowledgeWorks Global Ltd.

Contents

List of figures

List of tables

Acknowledgments

Plenty of people have contributed to this book and an unforgettable PhD time. Nevertheless, the responsibility for remaining errors and flaws is fully mine

To begin with, I want to thank the Hans Boeckler Foundation (HBS) for funding my thesis and the framework program it offered.

Furthermore, I thank the Bremen International Graduate School of Social Sciences (BIGSSS) for complementary funding, infrastructure, training, and intellectual exchange. I appreciated the institution for its collegiality but also for the friendly companionship – in particular of Katharina Bürkin, Ulrike Ehrlich, Saipira Fürstenberg, Jean-Yves Gerlitz, Michelle Hollman, Nepomuk Hurch, Andreas Katsikidis, Katharina Klug, Nora Waitkus, and the regular lunch break suspects.

My supervisors, Karin Gottschall, Heinz Rothgang, and Ian Greer naturally deserve a special mention. I thank Karin for following my project closely and supervising it conscientiously while also keeping an eye on the professional life afterward. Heinz contributed to the success of this project with his vast expertise on the health sector and his positive spirit. I thank Ian for having paved the path to this research field, for his comments, a very fruitful collaboration, as well as a research stay at the University of Greenwich.

Moreover, I am thankful to the University of Greenwich for accommodating me during my fieldwork. Here I met Geneviève Coderre-LaPalme and Nick Krachler, who I want to thank for extremely motivating academic exchange and collaboration.

For generous and useful comments at earlier stages of this project, I thank many (former) members of the BIGSSS faculty and other senior researchers I met during summer schools and research stays. I was also happy meeting many young researchers during my time in Oldenburg, Vienna, Paris, and London, and through other research activities, who made "networking" an enjoyable exercise.

I also want to express my deep gratitude to all interviewees for their precious time, honesty, and dedication.

I thank my close and dearest friends who reminded me of the world outside of academia and put things into perspective. Last, but not least, I thank my parents, sister and brother for their love, strong cohesion and sense of humour in difficult times. I thank my parents for everything they have given and taught me, their assurance to never let me down while letting me go my own way.

List of abbreviations

1199SEIU	*United Healthcare Workers East, Service Employees International Union*
AfC	*Agenda for Change – National Terms and Conditions of Employment*
BMA	*British Medical Association*
CCGs	*Clinical Commissioning Groups*
CFM	*Charité Facility Management*
DIVI	*Deutsche Interdisziplinäre Vereinigung für Intensiv- und Notfallmedizin e.V./German Interdisciplinary Association for Intensive and Emergency Medicine*
DKG	*Deutsche Krankenhausgesellschaft/German Hospital Federation*
DKV	*Deutsches Krankenhausverzeichnis/German Hospital Register*
DRGs	*Diagnosis-related groups*
FDP	*Freie Demokratische Partei/German Liberal Party*
FFL	*Fighting From Local*
GMB	*General, Municipal, Boilermakers, and Allied Trade Union*
GmbH	*Gemeinschaft mit Beschränkter Haftung/Company with Limited Liability*
GSTT	*Guy's and St. Thomas' NHS Trust*
HMO	*Health Maintenance Organization*
HSCA	*Health and Social Care Act*
KONP	*Keep our NHS Public*
MPs	*Members of Parliament, Members of Parliament*
NHS	*National Health Service*
NICE	*National Institute for Health and Care Excellence's guidance*
NUH	*Nottingham University Hospital*
NYSNA	*New York State Nurses Association*
ÖTV	*Gewerkschaft öffentliche Dienste, Transport und Verkehr/Public Sector Union*
PFI	*Private Finance Initiative*
PoN	*Protect our NHS*
RCN	*Royal College of Nursing*
RNs	*Registered Nurses*
SOU	*Strategic Organizing Unit*

SSA	*Safe Staffing Alliance*
TdL	*Tarifgemeinschaft deutscher Länder/Bargaining Union of the Federal States*
TUC	*Trade Union Congress*
TUPE	*Transfer of Undertakings (Protection of Employment) Regulations*
TVöD	*Tarifvertrag des öffentlichen Diensts/Public Sector Collective Agreement*
VdÄÄ	*Verein Demokratischer Ärztinnen und Ärzte/Association of Democratic Doctors*
ver.di	*Vereinte Dienstleistungsgewerkschaft/United Services Union*
VKA	*Vereinigung Kommunaler Arbeitgeber/Association of Local Government Employers*
VoC	*Varieties of Capitalism*
VSG	*Vivantes Service GmbH*

1 Marketization trends and trade unions in the health sectors

1.1 Introduction

The health sector is one of the most important pillars of mature welfare states. It deals with people in their most vulnerable conditions and is therefore a particularly sensitive activity. Yet, health sectors are not organized primarily around the patients' well-being but following economic principles, directed at cost containment and profit-making. Economic activity is widespread and ever increasing. Work in this sector is increasingly guided by economic incentives (Wehkamp and Naegler 2017). These detrimental incentives result in high costs not only for patients but also for employees in the sector. Since personnel costs clearly represent the largest share of health expenditure (Glassner, Pernicka, and Dittmar 2015, 67), they are usually the first target of cost cuts. Additionally, restructuring of work, business forms, and ownership are measures to lower costs, increase "productivity", and profits (see, e.g., Klenk 2011). As a consequence, employees suffer from insufficient staffing and work intensification that in turn inhibits them from performing their work properly and has clearly negative effects on patients' healthcare (see, e.g., Aiken et al. 2014). Employees in the health sector are torn between patients' well-being, their professional ethic, and their interests as employees (Chadwick and Thompson 2000). This makes the health sector a difficult field for trade unions to organize. However, it is an increasingly important sector for trade unions to organize in: Healthcare needs are increasing, the sector is expanding, marketization is advancing, and work intensification is growing.

Trade unions are one of the few actors opposing economization of the health sector and profit-making from the ill-being of patients. They have responded with a variety of different strategies to contain marketization and ease working conditions of employees. However, their success in the past was often limited. On the one hand, they were confronted with a strong political will of economization and austerity. However, on the other hand, trade unions did not always pursue their aims with the appropriate means. They often acted regardless of the special character of the sector, its marketization trends, or local-level resources. This book provides a differentiated assessment of macro-institutional framework conditions of healthcare marketization and a detailed analysis of local-level trade union resources, capabilities, and their fit with trade union strategies. How can trade unions in the healthcare sector (successfully) respond to marketization processes, and what are the determinants of their strategies?

To answer this question, in this chapter I will first present basic information on the health sectors and marketization trends, as well as the research program. In Chapter 2, I will assess theoretical approaches to the study of trade union strategies, considering local-level resources and capabilities, as well as the sector-specific institutional framework in times of marketization. The theoretical model will then be applied to the cases studied in Chapters 3 to 6. Finally, in Chapter 7, I will connect the findings of the four empirical chapters with one another and draw more general conclusions, suggest a refined model for the study of trade union strategies against marketization in the hospital sector, and discuss the contribution and limits of this research.

In this introductory chapter, I will now proceed with the provision of basic information on marketization, the specificities of the German and English health sectors, as well as their development over the last 30 to 40 years. I will then give a brief overview of trade unions in these sectors. Finally, I will present the research design and methods of this book.

1.1.1 General marketization trends

There are two main drivers that led to the general marketization and privatization trend in healthcare across developed capitalist countries. First, driven by aging societies, technological advancements, the need for new skills and qualifications, as well as the growing power of pharmaceutical and medical equipment industries, expenditure on health was increasing at the end of the 1980s. At the same time, the gross domestic product (GDP) growth slowed down, so that taxes and social contributions decreased due to unemployment, the rise of atypical jobs, and stagnation of wages. Therefore, countries felt an increased need for austerity. Further fueled by the EU's Stability and Growth Pact, countries started to try and contain costs also in the healthcare sector by setting incentives for competition and efficiency increases among providers (André and Hermann 2009, 130–133). This trend was intensified by the austerity measures implemented after the economic and financial crisis (Quaglio et al. 2013). The main instruments were the development of forms of privatization and marketization. In the health sector, this was done above all by means of budget setting and price controls based on the diagnosis-related groups (DRGs) (Stabile et al. 2013). Especially in the Southern European countries, this had a negative effect on health outcomes (Quaglio et al. 2013), most dramatically revealed during the Covid-19 pandemic in 2020.

Second, financial capital had become a major player and expected growing profits from the healthcare sector. Financial globalization further facilitated investment in healthcare sector assets (André and Hermann 2009, 130–133). Furthermore, private organizations were assumed to have higher efficiency, effectiveness, control of costs, and better quality (Maarse 2006, 1003).

As a consequence, the Organisation for Economic Co-operation and Development (OECD) countries have converged in healthcare regulation through the introduction of internal markets, competition, and negotiation, despite remaining differences in healthcare financing and other system-specific differences. Nevertheless, a shift from distinct types of health systems to mixed types can be observed (Rothgang et al. 2005).

Expenditure on health shows an increasing trend in both Germany and the UK, as well as in the OECD in general. Germany started with health expenditure of 9 per cent of its GDP in 1992, and after a steep increase in 2008 and a decline during the financial and economic crisis, it grew to 11.7 per cent by 2019. The UK increased its health expenditure more than Germany, starting at 5.9 per cent of its GDP in 1991, ever increasing until 2009, then stagnating and arriving at 10.3 per cent in 2019. The OECD average (data only available from 2003) followed the same trend but was well below the German and British expenses. However, also the OECD average expenditure on health increased from 7.0 to 8.8 per cent of the GDP from 2003 to 2019 (OECD 2020c) (see Figure 1.1).

While health expenditures increased, Rothgang et al. (2005) observed a decreasing share of *public* health expenditures in total health expenditure, leading to a partial shift from public to private financing. Even though total health expenditure increased, they coincided with other trends that moderate their potential positive effect on care quality, as well as on working conditions and pay for employees in the sector (see Section 1.2).

Nevertheless, it is worth noting that despite increases in health expenditures, experts nowadays agree that this cannot be referred to as a "cost explosion". This

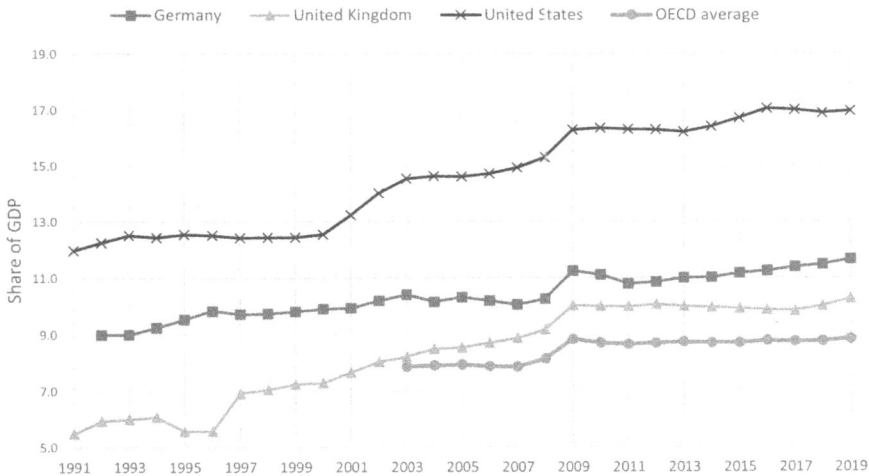

Figure 1.1 Current expenditure on health, all financing schemes, and providers.

Source: (OECD 2020c).

term was frequently used in Germany in the 1990s and served as justification for the introduction of the DRG reimbursement system. The new lump-sum payments for predefined treatment procedures were to replace the full-cost compensation and were supposed to contain costs. In fact, the DRGs had the opposite effect: instead of slowing down cost increases they became a driver. The share of statutory health insurance expenditure of the GDP was stable over decades. From 1980 to 2004, health insurance expenditure was about 6.1 to 6.5 per cent. After the introduction of the DRGs it increased to 7 per cent in 2017. The increase of statutory health insurance *contributions* from 13.2 per cent in 1994 to 15.5 per cent in 2011 was caused by increased unemployment and low-wage increases (IAQ 2019). Also, hospital expenses of the statutory health insurance increased since 1991. However, the increase was clearly steeper after the introduction of the DRGs (Statistisches Bundesamt 2020a).

In Germany, increasing expenditure was due to a higher number of patients treated, which is expressed in increased inpatient care discharges from 23,993 per 100,000 population in 2000 to 25,478 in 2017. In the UK, this number slightly declined from 13,566 to 13,144 (OECD 2020b). Treating a higher number of patients was facilitated through a shortened length of stay in Germany. The DRGs reimbursement system set the relevant incentives. While patients in Germany stayed in hospital for an average of 16.7 days in 1990 and 11.9 days in 2000, they were released after 8.9 days in 2017. Also, in the UK, the average length of patients' stays in hospitals decreased from 10.7 to 6.9 days between 2000 and 2017 (OECD 2020b). The increased workloads, however, were only partly compensated by an increase in healthcare employment. The number of health personnel employed in hospital (full-time equivalents) only slightly increased in both Germany and the UK during the same time period (OECD 2020a) (for more details see Section 1.2).

The mechanisms behind the described developments will be portrayed in more detail in the next sections, starting with a description of the two main concepts of privatization and marketization.

1.1.2 *Defining privatization and marketization*

Many of the reform trends in the two countries that will be outlined in Section 1.2 can be described with the terms privatization and marketization.

The term privatization is ideologically loaded and often used in ambiguous ways. "Privatization" is not a legal term, but an umbrella term for several forms of transfer of state tasks and responsibilities or their provision to a private legal entity. This can include a complete transfer of the task to the private sector, the provision of the task by a private provider, or the change of the provider's legal form. German administrative science distinguishes three main types of privatization that will be deployed in this book.

Formal privatization is characterized by the privatization of the organization, i.e., a change from a public to a private legal form and becoming subject to private law. The task as such remains in the public sector but is provided by

Table 1.1 Privatization types and characteristics

	Function	Provision	Ownership
Formal privatization	Public	Public, using private legal form	Public
Functional privatization	Public	Private	Public or Private
Material privatization	Private	Private	Private

Source: Author.

a private organizational form, e.g. a company with limited liability (GmbH). The majority ownership remains with the state. The aim of formal privatization is usually to release a company from its fiscal and administrative constraints and allow for more autonomy in day-to-day operations (Klenk 2011; Obinger, Schmitt, and Traub 2016). Functional privatization means that the state remains responsible for the task, but it commissions a private or other public entity to provide it. Public services are provided or funded by public entities, e.g., in commissioning, contracting out, outsourcing, and public private partnerships. The task can be commissioned either to a private provider, called external outsourcing, or to a public subsidiary, called internal outsourcing (Schulten and Böhlke 2009). It abolishes the principle that all public services are provided by the state, and creates an internal market in which public services buy support services from private providers or public subsidiaries (Givan and Bach 2007, 140). Material privatization describes the privatization of a state function. It is the partial or complete sale of public shares to private companies, the transfer of a task to the private sector where it is subjected to market competition. Material privatization is, thus, a shift of ownership from public to private (Obinger et al. 2016; see Table 1.1). Formal privatization will be discussed in Chapter 3 and functional and material privatization in Chapters 4 and 5.

Privatization is to be distinguished from marketization. However, the two processes affect one another and, in practice, often occur in combination.

Marketization can be understood as an increase in price-based competition at the level of the transaction.

> A fully marketized transaction is one with intense price-based competition, because actor choices are made purely on the basis of price, the good or service in question is standardized, exchanges are frequent, and competition is open to a wide range of participants.
>
> (Greer and Doellgast 2017, 195)

Whitfield (2006) defines marketization as "the process by which market forces are imposed in public services, which have traditionally been planned, delivered and financed by local and central government" (p. 4). In more detail, it includes five key elements: (1) the commodification of services and infrastructure, (2) the reorganization of work and jobs to maximize productivity and flexibility,

(3) restructuring the state for competition, (4) restructuring democratic accountability and user involvement, and (5) embedding business interests and promoting liberalization internationally (Whitfield 2006). Other authors add the organizational split between purchaser and provider, who transact money for services, as a key element (André and Hermann 2009, 136 f.; Greer and Doellgast 2017, 201).

At first sight, the term "marketization" seems to be an unsuitable description in the context of healthcare since prices are unified by the DRG reimbursement system. However, providing healthcare at a price that is lower than the reimbursed one can have similar effects to price-based competition. Hospitals have an incentive to provide services with least costs to reduce deficits, fund (unexpected) investments, or increase shareholder value (Klenk 2011, 264 f.). As Krachler and Greer (2015) have shown, active profit-making strategies of private providers in the English hospital sector do not consist of innovation in care as one might have expected, but of cost cutting and economies of scale, like in any other market. Private providers have a higher efficiency potential due to increased organizational autonomy, profit-oriented management and recruiting, lower wage costs and possibilities for staff reductions, as well as economies of scale (Klenk 2011, 266). Furthermore, in many hospitals new management practices have been implemented and administrations centralized to save costs, in addition to mass purchasing of supplies and equipment as well as sharing of expensive medical technology. In this way, hospitals were to mimic mainstream economic enterprises (Klenk 2011, 266). Also, Schwierz (2011) has shown how for the German hospital sector providers follow market mechanisms and adapt to increasing demands. Klenk (2011) observed the rise of the for-profit hospital industry in Germany through formal, functional, and material privatization of hospitals. Even not-for-profit providers in Germany that might be driven by a public goal must reserve assets for (unexpected) investments, and many not-for-profit as well as for-profit hospitals consistently show an annual surplus. While not-for-profit hospitals are expected to reinvest their surpluses, for-profit hospitals will distribute them among their shareholders (Klenk 2011, 264 f.).

Greer and Doellgast (2017) distinguish four forms of marketization: internationalization of trade, vertical disintegration, international labor migration, and labor market liberalization. These forms of marketization can be induced by the above-described forms of privatization: Formal privatization allows hospitals to act as an economic entity and to borrow money on the financial markets, thus increasing price-based or "cost-based" competition. Further, formal privatization is usually closely connected to other forms of privatization that increase marketization as well: Functional privatization leads to full exposure of services to market competition. When services are contracted-out, usually the cheapest bidder will be commissioned. In this case, competition is widening, an increased number of providers can participate in the market. Both national and multinational providers can theoretically enter the market. This has happened with respect to support services in both countries studied, as well as in medical services commissioning in England. When a hospital is sold off, private for-profit providers start extracting profits. The pursuit of profits sets off a process of intensified competition. Providers compete for patients and specialize in treatment procedures (Schwierz 2011; Krachler and Greer 2015). Furthermore, as in the case of functional privatization, hospital sell-offs increase the number of market participants by opening the provision to private providers, both nationally and internationally.

As the examples given above illustrate, privatization and marketization are two interlinked processes. Marketization can lead to privatization and vice versa. In this book, the terms will not be used interchangeably, but their interactive effect will be stressed. Thus, when speaking of privatization, there will usually be a marketization process connected to it and vice versa.

1.1.3 Relevance of the topic

Studying marketization in the health sector appears to be a worthwhile effort given that it is one of the sectors most exposed to marketization and privatization (Grimshaw et al. 2007, 609). German hospitals have been privatized at an unprecedentedly high rate in comparison to any other country (Böhlke, Greer, and Schulten 2011).

Since healthcare is also a labor-intensive sector, in which wages can account for 60 to 85 per cent of total operating expenses (Schwartz 2001, 28; Glassner, Pernicka, and Dittmar 2015, 67) and cost containment is the aim of marketization, the result is usually pressure on employees, deteriorating working conditions and lower pay. Therefore, especially in times of marketization, unions should have an interest in opposing marketization and/or containing its effects on workers.

The effects on the workforce can be illustrated using the example of nurses. In international comparison, nurses in Germany and the UK are facing work intensification and are on average responsible for considerably more patients than in other countries of the EU (Aiken et al. 2011). Subsequently, dissatisfaction among nurses is very high, overtime is very common (Griffiths et al. 2014), and around 40 per cent of nurses in Germany and England indicated their intention to leave the job within one year (Aiken et al. 2013, 147). This dissatisfaction and intention to leave the job are not only alarming in terms of working conditions but are also with respect to the problem of staff shortages (Kuehn 2007, 10; Blum et al. 2016). The introduction of the Californian staffing ratios has proven to improve work satisfaction (Aiken et al. 2010), which could encourage nurses working part-time to cope with the high workloads to return to full-time work or nurses who left the job to re-enter the job.

Finally, marketization has a strong effect on care quality, as shown by studies on outsourcing support services and the increase in hospital-acquired infections (Lethbridge 2012) or the relation of nurse staffing on patient mortality or nurses' workloads and adverse care effects (Aiken et al. 2011; Schreyögg 2016). Not least because of these effects, public interest in healthcare issues is high and more than 95 per cent of respondents in both Germany and Great Britain preferred public provision of healthcare (ISSP Research Group 2008).

After having assessed the relevance of the topic, I will discuss the distinct healthcare systems and how they create similar pressures for marketization and privatization, even though major differences in the role of the state with regard to healthcare financing remain.

1.2 Distinct healthcare systems, universal phenomena of marketization

This section will portray the characteristics of the British and German healthcare systems and will give a detailed analysis of policies of the last 30–40 years that led to the different forms of privatization and marketization in the sector.

Even though the role of the state in the funding and provision of health services differs in the German social insurance type and the British NHS type, reforms unfold comparative competitive pressure for hospitals and subsequently for workers and unions.

1.2.1 British hospital sector

The British healthcare system is a model of Beveridge-style welfare provision and belongs to the type National Health Service (NHS) in which regulation, financing, and provision are governed (mainly) by the state, funded by taxes and free for all citizens at the point of delivery (Böhm et al. 2013, 264 f.). It is an exception to Esping-Andersen's (1999) observation that the British welfare state diverged from the Nordic welfare states from the 1970s on, by failing to "supplement modest flat-rate benefits with a guarantee of adequate income replacement", which promoted "a gradual privatization that was no doubt accelerated by concerted deregulation [and] more targeting" (p. 87). The NHS remains state-dominated in funding, provision, and regulation, even in England, where marketization has gone furthest (Greer 2004). Services are overwhelmingly tax-funded (82.8 per cent in 2011/2012) (Krachler and Greer 2015), purchased by the state on behalf of citizens, with universal coverage.

The NHS was established in 1948. Its introduction has to be seen in the context of strong national solidarity after the Second World War (Baggott 2004, 86 ff.) which today is still present in the "collective mind" (Halbwachs 1985). This context helps to explain the importance and legitimacy that the public attributes to the NHS despite a general preference for more liberal social policies in other areas (Glassner, Pernicka, and Dittmar 2015, 10).

Health expenditure in the UK accounts for 10.3 per cent of the GDP (2019) (OECD 2020c). Operating costs are reimbursed following a DRG system. State funding accounts for 83.5 per cent of health expenditure, while 2.8 per cent of the total health expenditure was covered by private medical insurance, 9.3 per cent by out-of-pocket payments and 5 per cent from other forms of private expenditure (2015) (Cylus et al. 2015, xix). In contrast to Germany with 8 hospital beds per 1,000 population (2017), the, the UK has a particularly low number of hospital beds: 2.54 per 1,000 population (2019) (OECD 2020a).

Also, in contrast to Germany and despite numerous political attempts to increase private sector participation in healthcare, private sector involvement is very limited. Profit-making in the sector is difficult due to state dominance of funding and provision, a top-down squeeze on prices, uncertainty in market rules, and a high politicization of private provision of healthcare (Krachler and Greer 2015, 219 f.). Only 12.3 per cent of secondary care expenditure is paid to private providers (2012) (Krachler and Greer 2015, 216). The share of private hospital acute care beds only amounted to 6.5 per cent in England (2007) (Boyle 2011, 174). The share of hospital beds in public ownership exceeds 90 per cent in the UK (Böhm et al. 2013, 265).

Marketization in the British hospital sector has a long history and was pursued regardless of the political orientation of the governments. Trade unions did not manage to prevent reforms on the national level but succeeded at mediating some of their effects. The review of marketization reforms will focus on England since it covers 85 per cent of the UK population and most marketization processes have taken place there (Heins and Parry 2011, 382).[1] Marketization in England has taken different forms, starting with contracting out of ancillary services, continuing with increased entrepreneurial freedoms of NHS trusts, the creation of an internal market, and finally increased participation of private providers in financing infrastructure and provision of medical services.

The Conservative government (1979–1997) started marketization of the hospital sector with a reorganization of the general management in the NHS, in order to increase efficiency as suggested by the Griffith report, and with the introduction of competitive tendering for domestic, catering, and laundry services in 1983 (Griffiths 1983; Klein 2006, 46 ff., 128 ff.) (for more detailed information on outsourcing of support services in the NHS see Section 1.2.1.2 and Chapter 4).

At the beginning of the 1990s, the Conservative government continued its marketization reforms with the introduction of an internal quasi-market. Health authorities no longer provided and remunerated medical services, but general practitioners (GPs) and District Health Authorities (DHAs) became purchasers buying services from the providing hospitals for their patients (Pond 2006, 5). Hospitals in turn became self-governing NHS trusts which created the possibility of competition for service provision (Boyle 2011, 109 ff.). Nevertheless, the internal market at that time was highly restricted since trusts had to return surpluses to the government, were highly regulated, were not allowed to compete on prices, and providers could not be changed without consulting the Department of Health (Propper and Bartlett 1997, 17 ff.).

The third important marketization reform of the Conservative government was the Private Finance Initiative (PFI), a public-private partnership scheme introduced in 1992. To keep hospital expenditures off government accounts (Lethbridge 2012, 10), the Conservative government gave the trusts the possibility to hand over the tasks of borrowing money, designing and building new buildings to private consortiums. The private partners then not only design, build, and finance new buildings but also operate them, i.e., run auxiliary services such as catering, cleaning, portering and security (Pond 2006, 12). PFI contracts are marked by very long duration of usually 30 to 60 years (Lethbridge 2012) and annual borrowing fees that tend to put the trusts under severe financial pressure (Hellowell 2015). This policy was continued and extensively used by the New Labour government from 1997 to 2010 (Grimshaw, Vincent, and Willmott 2002).

New Labour further intensified performance management by means of its NHS plan, implemented from 2000 to 2002, but at the same time increased the average annual NHS funding by 6 per cent (Department of Health 2000, 451, Tailby 2012). With its NHS plan, it also introduced Independent Sector Treatment Centres (ISTCs), which are owned and run by private companies. Their purpose was to increase capacities, to reduce waiting lists for hospital treatments, to increase competition, and to stimulate innovation (Bishop and Waring 2011). However, in 2009, there were merely 34 ISTCs, accounting for only 1.79 per cent of elective care activities of the NHS in 2007/2008 (Naylor and Gregory 2009, 2 f.).

Shortly after, in 2003, New Labour introduced the legal form of NHS foundation trusts, as well as the payment by results reimbursement system through the Health and Social Care (Community Health and Standards) Act. Foundation trusts are owned by the state, but are more autonomous than the NHS trusts since they make their own financial decisions, may borrow from any lender, can establish profit-oriented business branches, receive up to 49 per cent of their total income from private patients, and can keep surpluses (but have to reinvest them) (Pollock et al. 2003, 21 f.; Leys and Player 2011) (for more information on foundation trusts and formal privatization see Section 1.2.1.1 and Chapter 3).

Payment by results is a form of activity-based funding, based on so-called healthcare resource groups. It is the British equivalent to the DRGs reimbursement system. It replaced the system of annual block contracts, in which the Department of Health and hospitals agreed on a sum of money for a given amount of activity, irrespective of the work actually carried out. The DRG system established standard tariffs for medical treatment procedures, regardless of the actual costs or the provider. However, many activities are excluded from this system (Pond 2006, 112, 115) compared to the DRG system in Germany.

The most recent major reform of the NHS and the core of the Conservative-led coalition government's health policy was adopted in 2012 with the Health and Social Care Act (HSCA). It further increased competition and private sector participation by stipulating the commissioning of medical services by Clinical Commissioning Groups (CCGs) (Davies 2013) (also see Section 1.2.1.3 for more information on commissioning of clinical services).

However, as mentioned in the previous section, the effects of the above-described policies to increase private sector involvement in healthcare were not as strong as expected. In 2012, secondary care expenses for private providers barely exceeded 12 per cent (Krachler and Greer 2015, 216), and more than 90 per cent of hospital beds remained in public ownership in the UK (Böhm et al. 2013,

265). Also, hospital income from private patients in NHS England has barely increased since the HSCA 2012 lifted the cap on the delivery of private services for foundation trusts (Watt 2014). Nevertheless, expenditure on private providers has increased significantly throughout the last years (Boyle 2011, 113). While in 2006, the NHS paid £5.6bn to non-NHS providers of care, this sum already increased to £8.7bn in 2011/2012 (Arora et al. 2013, 4) and amounted to over £10bn in 2013/2014 (King's Fund 2014, 6).

An important factor that accelerates marketization in this sector is the strong cost pressure induced by the government's austerity measures. According to these policies, 18.5 per cent of the NHS budged had to be cut by 2015 (Krachler and Greer 2015, 217). Consequently, since 2013, all trusts are required to deliver efficiency savings of 4 per cent per year (National Audit Office 2014a).

In the following section, the three main forms of marketization studied in this book and its main effect – understaffing – will be outlined for England.

1.2.1.1 Corporatization

Inspired by the Spanish "fundaciónes sanitarias", which are hospitals of the Spanish NHS, but managed by a private company, in 2003 the Labour Minister of Health, Alan Milburn, introduced the legal form of NHS foundation trusts through the Health and Social Care (Community Health and Standards) Act. Unlike in Spain, originally, foundation trusts were not to be managed by private companies but were to be given the same financial and operational freedom (Leys and Player 2011, 20 f.).

Foundation trusts operate like private businesses with limited liability, with a board of directors and ownership of their assets. Consequently, they have the freedom to sell any assets, borrow on the private financial market, enter into joint ventures with private companies, and set their own terms of employment. What distinguishes them from private companies is that they can only sell assets with the permission of the Secretary of State, they cannot make profits for shareholders, and they cannot earn more than 49 per cent of their total income from private patients (Leys and Player 2011, 21 f.). Foundation trusts are accountable to two independent regulators; their financial performance is regulated by Monitor, their healthcare services by the Care Quality Commission (National Audit Office 2011). Since foundation trusts are managed independently of the government, the transformation into a foundation trust can be classified as formal privatization (Pollock 2003).

Trusts can only become foundation trusts if judged financially sustainable, well-led, and locally accountable, as well as having good governance arrangements ensuring care quality by Monitor, the independent and unelected (Pollock 2003) regulator, sponsored by the government. Monitor assesses NHS trusts for foundation trust status and intervenes when trusts are in significant breach of their regulatory conditions, i.e., financial deficits or poor quality of care (National Audit Office 2014b).

Initially, all NHS trusts should have been in a position to apply for foundation trust status by 2008. This deadline was extended to 2014 and beyond for exceptional cases. Especially the trusts in London were struggling to achieve foundation trust status (National Audit Office 2011). By the end of 2013, the NHS England had 147 foundation trusts and 98 NHS trusts that had not yet attained foundation trust status (National Audit Office 2014b). Since 2013, all trusts are required to deliver efficiency savings of four per cent per year (National Audit Office 2014a). This magnifies the challenge to meet the requirement of financial sustainability for many trusts. The situation is even more difficult for trusts with PFI schemes. In 2011, 48 of 113 trusts applying for foundation trust status were unlikely to meet the financial standards set by Monitor. Among these 48 trusts, 22 had major PFI schemes. Out of these 22 trusts, 6 were not able to repay their debts and, together with other financial problems, were not financially viable (National Audit Office 2011).

Even though the NHS budget was in surplus from 2008 to 2014, foundation trusts have reported worse financial results, lower surpluses, higher values of fixed assets, and more indebtedness since 2008, when they were required to prepare their accounts according to the International Financial Reporting Standards. Roderick and Pollock (2014) suspect that deficits can also be reported to facilitate discontinuity of NHS services.

At the end of 2015, 12.7 per cent of all foundation trusts were rated at risk of failing to guarantee the continuity of their services by Monitor. 37.7 per cent were subject to enforcement action or under review due to poor governance and finance rating, of which eight were subject to special measures. One-third of the trusts were under regulatory action from Monitor since 2004, however, as many as 90 per cent of the trusts after 2013 (also see Tables 1.2–1.4).

Foundation trusts have an increased responsibility to generate surpluses for investments in services (Pollock 2003), but also have more possibilities at hand to balance their books and increase their profits than NHS trusts. The HSCA 2012 lifted the cap on the delivery of private services to 49 per cent for foundation trusts. This enables hospitals to give contracts to private companies to manage hospital pharmacies or restaurants. Furthermore, staff can be provided by private contractors (see Section 1.2.1.2), and clinical services can be subcontracted as well (Pollock 2003) (see Section 1.2.1.3). Some hospitals created entirely private

Table 1.2 Continuity of services rating

	1 – Most risk to fail	2	3	4 – Least risk to fail
No. of foundation trusts	19	17	42	72
Percentage	12.7%	11.3%	28%	48%

Source: Own database, generated from https://www.gov.uk/government/publications/nhs-foundation-trust-directory/nhs-foundation-trust-directory, accessed October 10, 2015. Total no. of foundation trusts: 150 (three trusts not rated).

Table 1.3 Governance rating

	Green No evident concerns	Red Subject to enforcement action	Under review Financial or governance concerns
No. of foundation trusts	94	38	19
Percentage	62.3%	25.2%	12.6%

Source: Own database, generated from https://www.gov.uk/government/publications/nhs-foundation-trust-directory/nhs-foundation-trust-directory, accessed October 10, 2015. Total no. of foundation trusts: 151 (two trusts newly authorized, no rating yet).

Table 1.4 Regulatory action

	No regulatory action	Regulatory action once	Regulatory action more than once	Further information requested
No. of foundation trusts	88	26	21	18
Percentage	57.5%	17.0%	13.7%	11.8%

Source: Own database, generated from https://www.gov.uk/government/publications/nhs-foundation-trust-directory/nhs-foundation-trust-directory, accessed October 10, 2015. Total no. of foundation trusts: 153.

outpatient facilities, and certain authors observed a rapid expansion of private patient services (Leys and Player 2011, 23; Roderick and Pollock 2014). However, the overall income from private patients in the NHS England remained well below 1 per cent of hospitals' total income (Watt 2014).

1.2.1.2 Outsourcing

Competitive tendering of NHS services has a long history (Pollock 2004). It was introduced in 1983 by the Conservative Health Minister Gerard Vaughan[2] to "release money for looking after patients" (Conservative Party 1983) and as part of a more generalized programme of efficiency savings. It coincided with the abolition of the Fair Wages Resolution, which used to oblige contractors providing public services to abide by the public sector wage rates (Cousins 1988, 219). This was regarded as the abandonment of the "model employer" approach of the state (Davies 2005, 15).

Since support services in the hospital sector are labor intensive, cost savings are mainly achieved by intensifying work, reducing pay, and lowering standards in working conditions. Therefore, the regulation of working conditions and pay became a major issue for unions.

While the transfer was well regulated in the past, it had been diluted in more recent times: The conditions under which public employees could transfer to private contractors were stipulated in the Transfer of Undertakings (Protection of Employment) Regulations (TUPE) (SI 1981/1794), which were the British implementation of the European Union Business Transfer Directive (Council Directive 77/187/EEC of February 14, 1977) introduced in 1981. TUPE regulations stated that any person who had been employed by the old employer automatically retained their previous terms and conditions when they became employed by the new employer. Collective agreements that had been valid with the old employer were inherited as well. The same held true for union recognition. Trade unions or employee representatives were also to be notified when a contract was awarded and were to be consulted if measures related to the transfer could affect employees. Employees were protected against dismissal for any reasons connected to the transfer. Pensions were excluded from any transfer.[3] The TUPE regulations applied when an undertaking was outsourced for the first time, but also when it was re-assigned to a new contractor. A precondition for the categorization as a transfer was that the service retained its identity and was carried on by the employee (UNISON 2014, 11 ff.). Public sector unions pursued successful cases in court in the 1980s and early 1990s that affirmed requirements under the TUPE. However, TUPE provisions retained ambiguities and possibilities for circumvention; for instance, varying conditions for transferred staff could be justified with economic, technical or organizational reasons (Lethbridge 2011, 72). Furthermore, they did not apply to staff hired after the transfer (Foster and Scott 1998, 143).

Finally, the TUPE regulations were updated in 2006 (SI 2006/246). The rights and obligations of the 1981 regulations remained in place, but were clarified at some points and rulings from case law were included (Department of Trade and Industry 2007). Furthermore, the TUPE regulations were amended by the Collective Redundancies and Transfer of Undertakings (Protection of Employment) (Amendment) Regulations 2014, which implemented the Acquired Rights Directive (ARD). This directive loosened TUPE regulations and today makes it easier to circumvent them, for instance, if activities carried out under a contractor are not "fundamentally the same", terms and conditions could change and dismissals would no longer be automatically unfair if the sole or principal reason is the transfer (ACAS 2014). As such, transferred contracts are no longer bound to any collective agreement developments, and the employer can seek agreement with the individual employee to change the terms and conditions incorporated in the collective agreement one year after the transfer if the *overall* terms are no less favorable than the current ones (UNISON 2014, 12).[4]

Differing terms and conditions applying to new recruits led to a two-tier workforce in subcontractor firms. In a report UNISON documented how new recruits earned considerably lower pay and other benefits than employees who transferred under TUPE regulations from the NHS to subcontractor firms. The New Labour government agreed to act and introduced, first in 2003, an initial version of the Code of Practice on Workforce Matters in Public Sector

Contracts, known as the two-tier code, that was also extended to the NHS in 2005 (Grimshaw 2009, 447; Tailby 2012, 454). This represented the largest achievement of trade unions under the New Labour government (Bach and Kessler 2012, 150). It was widely implemented in the NHS and extended the coverage of the NHS national agreements to privatized workers (Galetto, Marginson, and Spieser 2014). However, the two-tier code was withdrawn by the coalition government in 2010 and replaced with six Principles of Good Employment Practice. The principles *encourage* "fair and reasonable pay, terms and conditions", as well as consultation with trade unions on workforce training and development issues (Cabinet Office 2010a, 2010b). They are voluntary and "far less rigorous", according to UNISON. Therefore, the withdrawal of the two-tier code represents "a major threat" to TUPE protection after the transfer (UNISON 2014, 19).

Despite the above-described regulations, and probably due to the loopholes in them, competitive tendering is regarded as suitable for cost containment – politically convenient cost containment, since the outsourcing decision has to be made at the local level (Pollock 2004). However, despite anticipated cost savings, instead of a noticeably increased budget available for patient care, the government cut taxes. Furthermore, cost savings were overestimated, as a study focusing on the Scottish NHS revealed (Milne and Wright 2004). This might be due to increased administrative, monitoring and evaluation costs that accompany contracting out (Cousins 1988, 220). At the start, contracting out was effectively limited to catering, cleaning and laundry services (Davies 2005), but was regarded as an initial stage of a longer process of contracting out NHS services and the creation of public service "quasi-markets" (Le Grand 1991). While the Conservatives still limited contracting out to support services, the New Labour government extended it to clinical and pathology services in 2000 with its NHS Plan (Lethbridge 2012). Even though the Labour government made competitive tendering voluntary – instead of compulsory like before – and even though their rhetoric was less hostile and they made more public money available for investment (Grimshaw, Vincent, and Willmott 2002), the Labour government promoted competitive tendering, in particular through the increased use of the PFI schemes. As described above, the PFI allows trusts to receive private funding for public investments. In return, this usually includes the operation of facilities and provision of support services by the private partner (Lethbridge 2012, 4).

Up until the financial years 1982–1983 and 1983–1984, only 2 per cent of NHS England's expenditure on cleaning went to contractors and usually only concerned NHS offices (Davies 2005, 16 f.). Private contractors were also not very successful at winning bids in the 1980s. They won only 18 per cent of the contracts by 1987 (Cousins 1988, 220). UNISON estimated the extent of contracted out cleaning services to be at 30 per cent of NHS cleaning services in 2002, worth about £330m (Davies 2005, 16 f.).[5] A new market was created for private sector firms. Today this market is dominated by few and mostly foreign multinational companies. The top four companies that held about 51 per cent of the market (2003) were ISS, Compass, Sodexho, and Rentokil Initial. These companies usually do not only provide cleaning but hold multiservice contracts to benefit from economies of scale. The reliance on a small group of large multinational companies to provide essential support services, as well as a lack of accountability, is regarded as problematic by UNISON (Davies 2005, 16 f.).

Another downside to competitive tendering for support services, besides the cost savings that did not materialize to the extent proclaimed by the Conservatives, was a deterioration in care quality (Walness 2002). Even though support service workers' main task is not patient care, they are in contact with patients and make caring contributions. Isolating them from the healthcare team and intensifying their workload keeps ancillary service workers from making their contribution to patient care and, in consequence, also increases workloads for nurses. Furthermore, managers lose direct control over quality in the area of outsourced services (Cousins 1988, 223, 225). The deterioration in care quality was particularly striking with respect to cleaning. Cleaning plays an important role in reducing hospital infections, as shown in various studies (Lethbridge 2012). During the 1990s, there was a considerable increase in hospital acquired infections, such as MRSA (methicillin-resistant *Staphylococcus aureus*) and *C. difficile*. This was traced back to a lack of expertise and poor training of staff, as well as a lack of continuity between cleaners, clinical staff, managers, patients, and visitors where cleaning services are outsourced. This acted to the detriment of a shared sense of responsibility for cleanliness across the hospital. In addition, high staff turnover and sickness absences were a problem. This is why the devolved governments in Scotland, Wales, and Northern Ireland have abandoned outsourcing of cleaning (Givan and Bach 2007, 146). The need to act upon cleaning standards in the NHS was acknowledged by the government as well, which is reflected in reports on the reduction of hospital acquired infections (National Audit Office 2004).

1.2.1.3 Medical services commissioning

While public tendering of support services in the NHS has a long tradition, it did not concern clinical services until recent times and only a small share of medical services has been provided by the above-mentioned ISTCs. The HSCA 2012 of the Conservative-led government aimed to facilitate private sector participation in medical services provision. The Act introduced CCGs. These are made up mostly of GPs who are responsible for tendering out health services (Davies 2013). The HSCA was strongly opposed by unions through campaigns, but they could not prevent its introduction (Heins and Parry 2011, 391).

In contrast to Germany, no hospital in Britain was sold to a private provider. The closest England came to privatizing a hospital was in 2011, when the management and finance of a small, financially troubled hospital in Cambridgeshire, Hinchingbrooke, was contracted out to Circle UK (Scourfield

2016). Therefore, the commissioning of clinical services to private providers functions as an analytical equivalent to hospital privatizations in Germany in this book (see Chapter 5).

1.2.1.4 Understaffing

The reason for understaffing in England, as in most OECD countries, is mostly a politically induced constraint of health expenditure growth realized through the above-described marketization policies. Also in England, staffing is the largest category in healthcare expenditure, both with respect to operating expenses and direct care costs (Aiken et al. 2011; Aiken et al. 2014). Cost pressures and marketization policies mainly translate into understaffing through the replacement of nurses with healthcare assistants and incentives that shorten the average length of stay of patients.

The number of nurses in the UK has increased by 23 per cent between 2003 and 2013, with a short period of decline between 2008 and 2010. There has been an even bigger growth in the category of nursing auxiliaries and assistants, rising by 39 per cent between 2003 and 2013 (RCN 2014, 4). The former cuts in staffing numbers have been reversed as a response to the Francis Report that revealed the harmful effect of outsourcing and reductions in personnel on patients' well-being. The upward trend in nursing follows the recent critical focus on safe staffing levels in hospitals. However, hospital staff numbers were increased at the expense of community and mental health nursing. Higher salaries for lower Agenda for Change pay system bands were at the expense of a reduction in senior nursing posts. Furthermore, the growth has only been fueled by high workforce increases in work areas of paediatric and neonatal nursing. In all other areas, there has been a decline in the numbers of qualified nurses (RCN 2014, 14–18).

Consequently, and despite staff increases, a survey conducted between 2009 and 2010 revealed that, during day shifts, one nurse in England was, on average, responsible for 7.8 patients. This staffing level is still better than in Germany (9.9), but far worse than, e.g., in the Netherlands (4.8) or Norway (3.7) (Aiken et al. 2013, 148). Since the publication of the Francis Report that revealed considerable deficits in care quality in 2013, reporting of staffing levels was made a requirement for hospital trusts. The NHS Choices website shows the average performance of hospitals across all wards against their own planned staffing levels.[6] An analysis by the Health Service Journal of this data showed that 96 per cent of 223 NHS acute hospitals in England did not achieve their planned staffing levels during the day shifts, and also during night shifts, with 85 per cent fewer nurses covering the shifts than planned in October 2016 (quarter three of 2016–2017). Performance has decreased since quarter four of 2014–2015 (see Figure 1.2). At the same time, those hospitals that remained below their planned staffing levels for nurses had higher than planned staffing levels of lower qualified healthcare assistant staff, especially at night (Lintern 2017b).

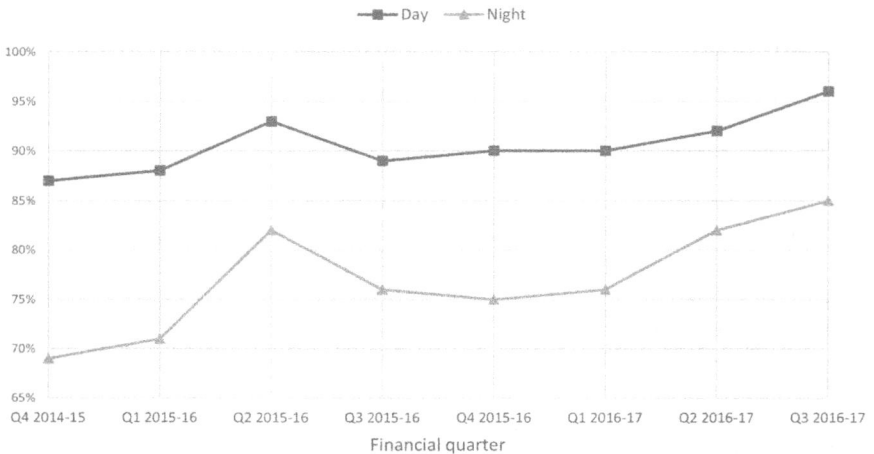

Figure 1.2 Hospitals failing to meet planned nurse staffing levels, England.

These trends even persist despite record recruitment of nurses in the acute sector. The RCN estimates that there are still 40,000 nursing vacancies in the service, and a survey carried out by the RCN also revealed that 9 out of 10 nursing leaders in the NHS are worried about their ability to recruit nurses due to the staff shortage (Lintern 2017a). This also contributes to a change in the skill mix supported by the government, with a high and growing share, as well as a more dominant role of healthcare assistants in Britain (Bach, Kessler, and Heron 2012). Only 57 per cent of caregivers are professional nurses in England, compared to 82 per cent in Germany (Aiken et al. 2013, 148). Figures for 2014 show that out of all nursing and caring professionals in Great Britain 35 per cent were nursing professionals, and 55 per cent were healthcare assistants (Eurostat 2016a). Even though it has to be noted that nurses in England are on average higher educated – 28 per cent of them holding a bachelor's degree while German nurses usually complete vocational training – the Netherlands, with comparably high rates of bachelor's degrees among nurses (32 per cent), show considerably higher staffing levels, with, on average, only 4.8 patients per registered nurse (Aiken et al. 2013, 145, 148). In addition, the average length of stay steadily decreased (OECD 2020a) (see Figure 1.3).

Subsequently, dissatisfaction among registered nurses in England is high. In general, 39 per cent of nurses are dissatisfied with their job, and 43 per cent intend to leave their current job within one year (Aiken et al. 2013, 147). However, in comparison, a relatively low share of nurses – 19 per cent – report poor quality patient care compared to 35 per cent in Germany. This share was only lower in Finland, Norway (both 13 per cent) and Ireland (11 per cent) (Aiken et al. 2013, 150). The reason might be that nurses in England compensate for bad staffing levels by working overtime. As many as 50 per cent of nurses reported to

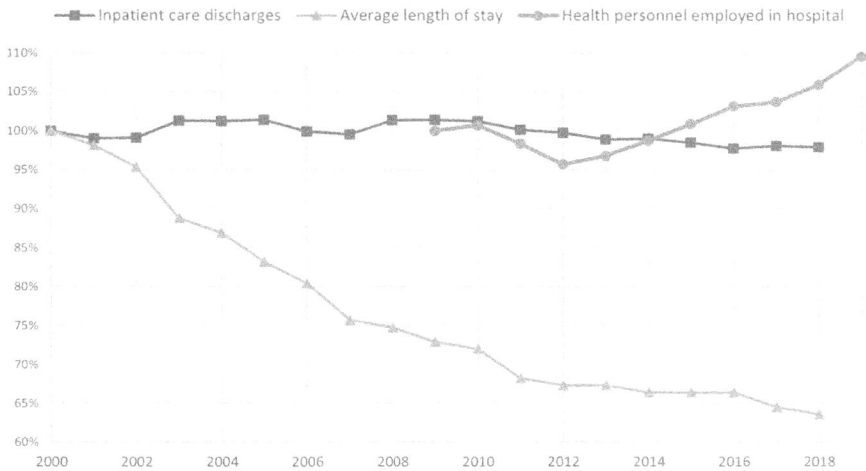

Figure 1.3 Work intensification in British hospitals.

have worked overtime (i.e., beyond their contracted hours) on their last shift, as opposed to 36 per cent in Germany (Griffiths et al. 2014).

1.2.1.5 Excursus: Understaffing trends in the USA

In Chapter 6, trade union struggles for staffing levels will be presented. Due to strong parallels of an US-American and a German case, an US-American case will be studied in Chapter 6. Therefore, this section also portrays understaffing trends in the USA.

In the US, the 1973 Health Maintenance Organization (HMO) Act marked the beginning of a period of increased use of market mechanisms. The 1973 Act provided grants to set up HMOs (Field 2014, 39) and it led to the growth of HMO-type organizations (White 2007). HMOs aim at containing costs by providing monthly per member premiums that have to cover all healthcare-related costs, having primary care physicians act as gatekeepers for care and restricting patient choice. In addition, policymakers have gradually outsourced the management of Medicaid and Medicare programmes to managed care insurers since the 1980s (Field 2014, 174) with the aim of inserting cost-reducing incentives into contractual relationships between insurers and providers. Managed care insurers administering public insurance programmes manage public funds but negotiate the price of provision down so that they are able to achieve profit margins for themselves, as well as cost savings for public insurance programmes.

Moreover, since the 1980s, alternatives to costly hospital inpatient care, such as urgent care centers and outpatient clinics, have proliferated (Scott et al. 2000). One factor in this proliferation was the introduction of DRGs in 1983. By fixing the price of reimbursements for services, DRGs provide guaranteed

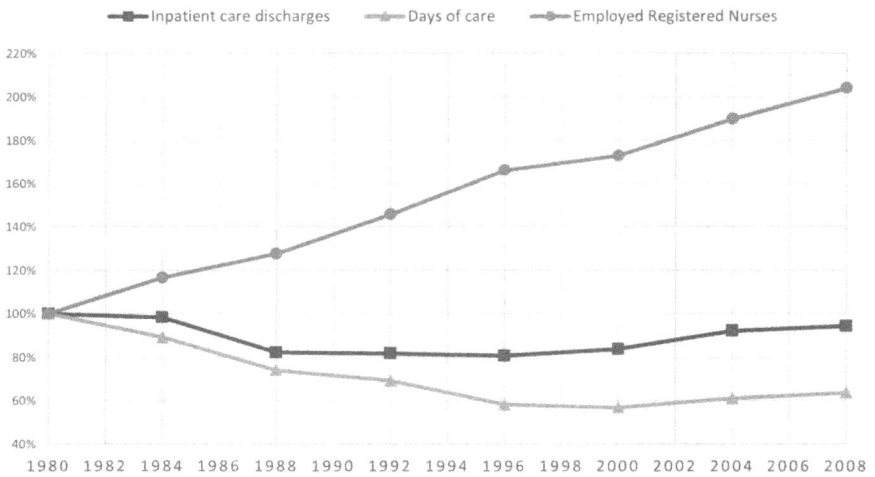

Figure 1.4 Work intensification in US-American hospitals.

revenues to hospitals, facilitating the growth in the number of for-profit hospital beds (Lutz and Gee 1998). Fixed prices also mean that providers have to lower their costs to achieve profit margins. Furthermore, since the 2010 Patient Care and Affordable Care Act, government agencies have begun to develop payment schemes such as Medicare Shared Savings that reward and penalize providers according to the quality of care they provide. This is leading to the increased establishment and usage of preventative care and ambulatory facilities (Blumenthal, Abrams, and Nuzum 2015). Alternatives to classic, more costly inpatient hospital care, such as HMOs, urgent care centers, and outpatient facilities, as well as managed care organizations and for-profit providers, have increased cost pressures in US healthcare (Clark et al. 2001).

In addition, in the US, the number of patients treated increased while the length of stay decreased; thus, nurses have to see more and sicker patients at the same time (Lafer 2005; Moody 2014). The fact that lengths of stay have been reduced while the number of discharges increased from 2000 onwards indicates this increase in workloads (U.S. Department of Health and Human Services 2010, 2008) (see Figure 1.4).

1.2.2 German hospital sector

The German healthcare system belongs to the Social Health Insurance type, with strong societal actors who play a dominant role in regulation and financing. Delivery of health services is typically on a private for-profit basis (Böhm et al. 2013, 265 f.).

Operating costs in German hospitals are funded following the DRG system by the health insurance funds, which are organized as membership-based, self-regulated organizations of payers and providers. The financing of infrastructure and hospital planning lies mainly in the responsibility of the German federal states. Since the early 1990s, hospital financing by the states has declined, which has forced hospitals to finance infrastructure from their operational business revenues (Augurzky, Krolop, and Schmidt 2010, 14 f.). This led to a yearly investment backlog of about €3bn and put hospitals under strong cost pressures

Statutory health insurance in Germany is compulsory for employees (as long as they do not exceed a certain income threshold), but they can freely choose which health insurance fund they want to join. Both employees and employers pay contributions which depend on gross income (Busse and Riesberg 2005, 30, 70, 74). About 89 per cent of Germans are covered by statutory health insurance, only about 11 per cent are privately insured (Gerlinger 2014, 36). Statutory health insurance covered 58.1 per cent of healthcare expenses in 2015 (Statistisches Bundesamt 2017).

Typical for Social Health Insurance healthcare systems, German hospitals are and were always owned by various private for-profit, private not-for-profit, and public providers. Over the past 30 years, the share of hospitals in private-for-profit ownership increased while public ownership dropped (also see Section 1.2.2.1). In EU-wide comparison, Germany has the largest share of privately provided hospital beds (2014) (Eurostat 2016b).

The DRG system was supposed to reduce excess capacities, i.e., to reduce the number of hospitals (Schwierz 2011). The number of hospitals decreased between 1991 and 2018 by 20.2 per cent and the number of beds by 25.1 per cent (Statistisches Bundesamt 2020b). However, with private providers buying formerly public hospitals despite low demand (Klenk 2011), Germany sustained the highest number of hospital beds relative to population size in the EU (8 beds per 1,000 inhabitants in 2017) (OECD 2020a).

In contrast to the British hospital sector, in the German hospital sector marketization and privatization were not driven by a variety of government policies, but rather indirectly, mainly due to a change in the reimbursement system and declining infrastructure investments by the states.

The most crucial reform in the hospital sector was the decoupling of hospital payments from the actual costs of provision that started in 1993. The Health Care Structure Act changed the financing system from full-cost coverage to a system of capped hospital budgets. The hospital reimbursement system was changed in 1996 from a per diem system to a mixed system of per diem and case fees. In 2003, the hospital reimbursement system was changed to the DRG system (see, e.g., Simon 2007a, 50 ff.). The DRG reimbursement system no longer guaranteed full-cost compensation; hospitals only receive lump-sum payments for pre-defined treatment procedures. In 2018, 29 per cent of German hospitals recorded an annual loss out of which 13 per cent had an increased risk of insolvency (Augurzky et al. 2020). This makes privatization attractive for public authorities as it reduces debt and discharges them of the duty to make further investments. Private hospitals have a competitive advantage in terms of being able to access private capital markets for investments more easily; they can use synergy and scale effects from the organization of their operational business in several hospitals. Furthermore, they are not covered by public sector collective agreements (Schulten 2006, 10).

Nowadays, DRGs in Germany are highly debated. There is substantial criticism that the DRGs were a driver of healthcare costs. They set incentives for hospitals to perform lucrative but medically unnecessary treatments (Augurzky 2012). The most prominent examples are knee and hip replacements that are carried out more frequently in Germany than in any other OECD country (OECD 2019). At the same time, healthcare services that are more difficult to plan and require more personnel such as paediatric and obstetric services are vastly undersupplied. Therefore, many stakeholders demand the (partly) replacement of the DRGs and return to full-cost coverage. For a detailed assessment of the shortcomings of the DRG system in Germany see Simon (2020).

The second driver of marketization was the issue of a declining state financing of hospitals prevalent since the early 1990s. The lack of funding increases put pressure on hospitals due to the fact that – even though it contravenes the law – they have to finance investments from their operational business revenues (Augurzky, Krolop, and Schmidt 2010, 14 f.).

In order to deal with increasing cost pressures, hospitals sought to reduce costs and to increase efficiency by means of outsourcing (Simon 2007b, 41–46) and changes in legal form to increase their economic flexibility and reduce costs. Accordingly, the share of public hospitals in private legal form increased steadily. However, costs per case in public corporatized hospitals are still higher than in private hospitals and corporatization is often a precondition for a later privatization (Schulten 2006, 8). In the same way, the main reason for outsourcing in Germany is the potential for cost reductions. However, quality improvements and material cost reductions often did not materialize as expected. Since corporatization and outsourcing were not yielding the expected results, they were often followed by privatization of hospitals. Although there have been no explicit privatization policies, the overall hospital sector economization increased the share of hospitals in private for-profit ownership. The three forms of privatization will be described in more detail in the following sections.

1.2.2.1 Corporatization

Corporatization in Germany was mainly driven by cost pressures brought about by insufficient funding from states for infrastructure investments and changes in the reimbursement system. In 2004, more than 30 per cent of German hospitals were not able to finance their operational business (Deutsches Krankenhausinstitut 2005). Corporatization was attractive for public authorities since it reduces debt and discharges them of the duty to make further investments. Furthermore, it increases the economic autonomy of the hospital that is regarded as an important precondition for competitiveness (Schulten and Böhlke 2009, 102). The costs per case in corporatized public hospitals are

Table 1.5 Costs per treated case in public and private hospitals in euro

	Total costs per case	Personnel costs	Material costs
Public hospitals	5,712	3,439	2,129
In public legal form	7,396	4,461	2,773
In private legal form	4,579	2,751	1,696
Private not-for-profit	4,383	2,672	1,581
Private for-profit	4,523	2,617	1,770

Source: Statistisches Bundesamt (2015), own presentation.

significantly lower than in their counterparts in a public legal form (Statistisches Bundesamt 2015) (see Table 1.5). However, since the costs per case in public corporatized hospitals are still higher than in private hospitals, corporatization cannot be regarded as a sustainable alternative to privatization but rather as a precondition for a later sell-off (Schulten 2006, 8)

From 2002 to 2009, the share of public hospitals in public legal form dropped from 26.4 to 12.7 per cent, while the share of public hospitals in private legal form increased from 10.4 to 18.4 per cent. Until 2017, the shares remained relatively stable and arrived at 11.6 per cent of public hospitals in public legal form and 17.3 per cent of public hospitals in private legal form in 2017 (Statistisches Bundesamt 2020b).

1.2.2.2 Outsourcing

Outsourcing in Germany started in the 1990s and concerned primarily support services, such as laundry and sterilization services, or facility management. From the 2000s onwards, clinical services, such as radiology, radiotherapy, and internal medicine, were contracted out as well. The main reason for outsourcing in Germany is the potential for cost reductions of 10 to 40 per cent within the first two to five years, as well as potential profits and quality control (Schweizer and Bernhard 2009, 373).

Outsourcing support services supposedly gives public hospitals the possibility to focus on healthcare, increasing its quality. However, one of the disadvantages is higher transaction costs. This is one reason why outsourcing was not always yielding the expected cost reductions and 10 per cent of all hospitals insourced formerly outsourced services between 2008 and 2013 (Blum et al. 2013, 40 ff.).

Nevertheless, outsourcing is regarded as the best and least risky option to improve a hospital's budget. It necessitates only low investments and generates high income in relation to relatively low expenses, especially in the long term. In comparison to material privatization, public-private partnerships, as well as mergers and acquisitions, outsourcing is also suitable for relatively low investment needs (below €1m). Furthermore, health sector experts do not have ethical concerns about outsourcing (Schweizer and Bernhard 2009, 377 ff.).

Service subsidiaries are regarded as profitable if they are recognized as a single-entity for tax purposes ("umsatzsteuerliche Organschaft") and are exempted from value-added tax. Moreover, they can generate profits that can be transferred to the hospital. In addition, the hospital subsidiary companies are not bound by the health sector collective agreement, but can employ workers according to other sectors' collective agreements that are cheaper in the long term (in the short term, transferred workers' pay, terms, and conditions are protected (Franke 2007, 193 f.)). These transfer regulations are laid down in the German civil code (§ 613a BGB) and are comparable to the TUPE in Britain (see Section 1.2.1.2). Transferred employees are guaranteed their pay, terms and conditions for one year after the transfer, unless the new employer belongs to or joins another employer's association and is thus subject to a different collective agreement (§ 613a Abs. 1 BGB). Further, employees in Germany have the legal right to appeal against their transfer to another employer within one month of notification (§ 613a Abs. 6 BGB). Employers are not allowed to lay off employees because of the transfer. However, in practice, it is difficult to prove that the transfer is the reason for the redundancy.

By 2013, 66 per cent of the cleaning services, 80 per cent of the laundry services, 41 per cent of the catering services, and 53 per cent of the pharmacies of German hospitals were contracted out. Apart from these most commonly outsourced services, also services like laboratories, radiology or logistics were outsourced. Outsourcing was particularly prevalent in smaller hospitals with less than 600 beds. Between 2008 and 2013, only 37 per cent of large hospitals with more than 600 beds outsourced services, in contrast to 49 per cent of all German hospitals. The main reason for outsourcing is usually a reduction in personnel and material costs, but also desired increases in quality and flexibility. Quality improvements and material cost reductions only materialized in 51 per cent and 43 per cent of cases, respectively. The lack of significant quality improvements was the most common reason for insourcing of services (42 per cent). Other problems were difficulties in communication with the private provider, a lack of commitment of employees and high staff turnover. This is why 10 per cent of all hospitals insourced formerly outsourced services between 2008 and 2013 (Blum et al. 2013, 40 ff.).

Outsourcing of support services led to an increase in the fragmentation of collective bargaining. The sector is not only fragmented in terms of hospital ownership and occupational groups, but outsourced hospital support services are also usually not part of the public sector collective agreement. This led to the development of a core and peripheral workforce within hospitals. Only 10 to 20 per cent of the publicly owned support service subsidiaries are part of collective agreements at all. If covered by an alternative collective agreement, this is particularly unfavorable for support service workers since the differences to the public sector agreement are greatest in the lower wage brackets (Glassner, Pernicka, and Dittmar 2015, 41 f.). This leads to a growing divide between a shrinking organized core and a disorganized periphery workforce. It yields disruptive changes: jobs are moved to companies with weaker firm-level

agreements, no collective agreements or agreements belonging to another sector. Trade unions are forced to network across an increasing number of locations
and to coordinate a variety of weak, firm-level collective arrangements. This also
contributes to weaker and more divided works councils, as well as increasingly
complex firm, sectoral and occupational bargaining structures (Doellgast and
Greer 2007, 70 f., Holst 2013).

1.2.2.3 Privatization

When corporatization and outsourcing did not reduce costs as expected or
hospitals were still in deficit, they often led to privatization. Instead of explicit
privatization policies, general cost pressures in the sector also fueled the sell-off
of hospitals.

The first wave of privatizations took place in East Germany after reunification,
motivated by an ideological commitment of policymakers to private ownership
and market competition (Schulten 2006, Schwierz 2011). A second wave of
privatizations took place after the introduction of the DRGs. Privatization was
regarded as a solution by local governments to access private capital and relieve
the municipal budget of the investment backlog. The first privatization of state-
owned university hospitals in 2006 was regarded as a temporary occurrence. In
the same year, the first German hospital provider was taken over by a foreign
hospital company (Schulten 2006, 3). Three large for-profit chains, Asklepios,
Helios, and Sana, emerged to acquire financially troubled public hospitals, both
small and large.

Consequently, between 1991 and 2018, the share of private for-profit ownership increased from 15 to 38 per cent. The share of publicly owned hospitals
dropped from 46 to 29 per cent in the same time period. Private not-for-profit
hospital providers, e.g., churches are still present in the sector, but their share
also decreased from 39 per cent in 1991 to 34 per cent in 2018 (see Figure 1.5)
(Statistisches Bundesamt 2020b). Compared to other OECD countries, Germany
is among the countries with the highest share of hospitals in private-for-profit
ownership (see Figure 1.6).

Regarding the number of beds, the picture is slightly different because the
largest hospitals with the highest number of beds usually remained in public
ownership. In 2018, 48 per cent of hospital beds were in public ownership as
compared to 54.5 per cent in 2002. During the same time period, private not-
for-profit hospitals decreased their share of beds from 36.7 per cent to 32.9 per
cent, while private for-profit hospitals more than doubled their share of beds from
8.9 per cent in 2002 to 19.1 per cent in 2018 (Statistisches Bundesamt 2020b).

1.2.2.4 Understaffing

Insufficient funding from the states and changes in the reimbursement system to
DRGs did not only fuel different forms of marketization. Hospitals in Germany
also have responded to these cost pressures by increasing the number of patients

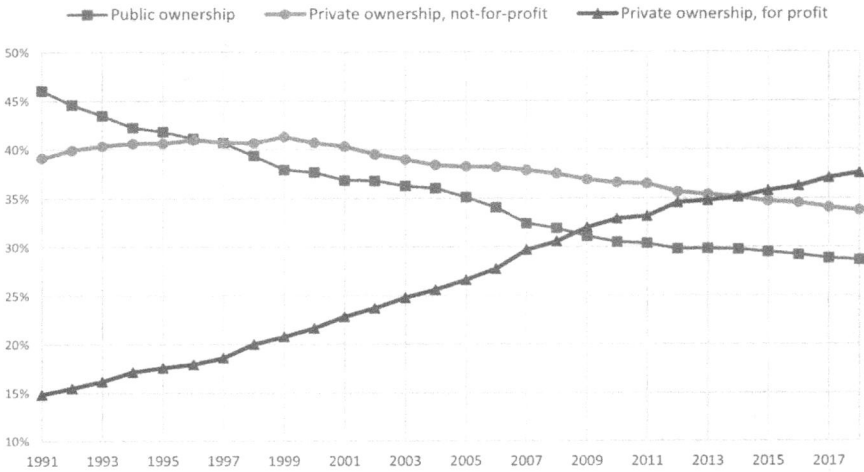

Figure 1.5 Ownership of German hospitals.

and reducing their length of stay while first reducing the number of health personnel and then increasing it under-proportionately in comparison to the number of patients (see Figure 1.7) (Statistisches Bundesamt 2020a). Especially for nurses, workloads increased since German hospital administrators have tended to increase the number of patients nurses see at the same time as patients were becoming sicker. Subsequently, nurses' workloads, expressed as cases per nurse, steadily increased, despite growing numbers of nurses from 2007 (see Figure 1.8).

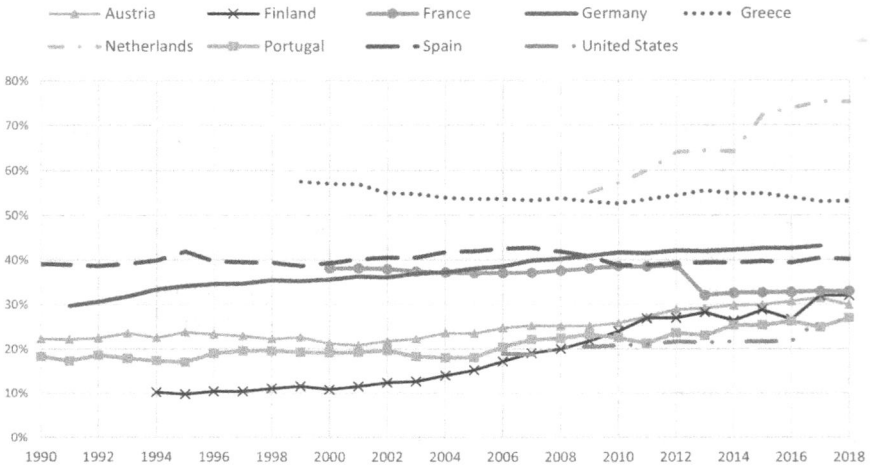

Figure 1.6 Private-for-profit ownership of hospitals, nine countries.

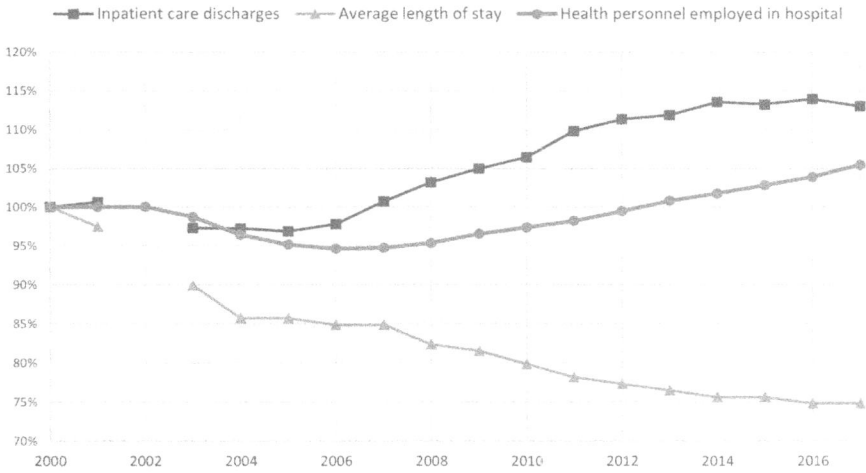

Figure 1.7 Work intensification in German hospitals.

The increased workloads fall to nurses, with one German nurse caring for 9.9 patients, on average, in 2010 (Aiken et al. 2011). A survey carried out in 224 hospitals by ver.di in 2015 showed that this situation is far worse during night shifts. In 55 per cent of cases, one nurse had to care for 25 patients. In intensive care units, nurses cared, on average, for 3.3 patients during the night, even though the German Interdisciplinary Association for Intensive and Emergency Medicine (DIVI) requests a professional standard of at least one nurse per two patients in intensive care units (ver.di 2015a). Accordingly, 37 per cent of nurses

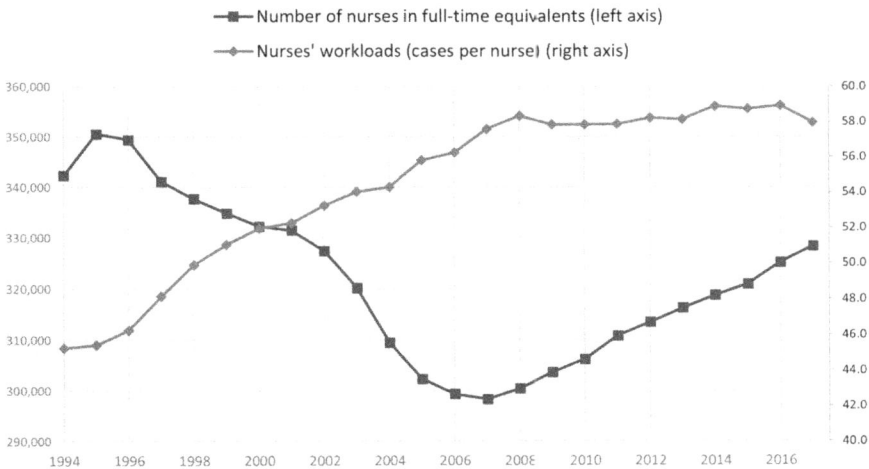

Figure 1.8 Number of nurses and nurses' workloads in German hospitals.

in Germany are dissatisfied with their jobs and 36 per cent also intend to leave the job within one year (Aiken et al. 2013, 147).

In comparison to England, the skill mix in Germany shows a higher-qualified staff with a share of 82 per cent of registered nurses among the caring and nursing personnel. However, it has to be noted, that the vast majority of nurses in Germany received vocational training whereas registered nurses in England need a bachelor's degree. At the same time, more healthcare *assistants* work in the NHS than in German hospitals (Aiken et al. 2013, 148). Anyways, the staffing shortage is also increasing in Germany, and one way to react is to change the skill and grade mix. A survey carried out by Blum et al. (2015, 41) shows (exemplarily for the surgical services) that 54 per cent of the responding hospitals assume that the number of healthcare assistants with only two years of vocational training will increase by 2020.

To conclude, the healthcare sector has witnessed considerable marketization that also had an effect on workers which makes it an important field for trade unions to organize in. The main unions and their responses to marketization will be presented in the next section.

1.3 Trade unions and marketization

After having assessed the different forms and effects of marketization and privatization in the two countries, the main actors studied in this book, the sector they are operating in, as well as their responses to marketization in this sector, mainly on the national level, will be described.

1.3.1 Employment relations and trade unions in the healthcare sectors

Usually, employment relations in Germany and England are considered to be of two distinct types. The coordinated and liberal market economies framework (Hall and Soskice 2001), however, does not adequately describe the situation in the public sector (Bach and Bordogna 2011). This holds true especially for the healthcare sector.

In contrast to the coordinated market economy type, in the German healthcare sector employment relations are unusually fragmented, and trade union density in this sector is above the national average. However, the trade union landscape is typically centralized and unions possess extensive co-determination rights.

The main collective actors in the health sector on the employees' side are the United Services Union 'ver.di 'and the Marburger Bund. Ver.di is the biggest union in the health sector. The union covers 385,063 employees in the health and social care sectors across all professions (ver.di 2019b, 74). Even though membership of ver.di as a whole is declining (from 2.8m in 2001 and 2.1m in 2009, to slightly below 2m in 2018; Deutscher Gewerkschaftsbund 2020), its membership in the health and social care sector has been increasing since 2011 when it covered 343,972 members. The increase in membership from 2015 to 2018 could be found first and foremost among trainees (+35.2 per cent), young employees up to 28 years (+16.6 per cent), and part-time workers (+7.1 per cent). 75 per cent of members in the health and care sector are women (ver.di 2019b, 75). Since 2011, ver.di's main focus in the hospital sector was the improvement of working conditions through demands for more personnel, especially an increase in the number of nurses, as well as organizing workers in outsourced support service companies (ver.di 2015b, 20–30, 2019b, 16–19, 24–36).

The second largest union is the Marburger Bund that exclusively organizes physicians. Its membership amounts to 127,000 physicians (Marburger Bund 2020). In German public hospitals, ver.di membership density is estimated at 23 per cent overall, with higher density levels in public hospitals and considerably lower, but varying levels, in private ones. The Marburger Bund's union density is estimated at 70 to 80 per cent among physicians (Glassner, Pernicka, and Dittmar 2015).[7] Members of ver.di pay a monthly membership fee of 1 per cent of their salary before tax. Ver.di's income from membership fees in the health and social care unit was €6.8m per month in 2018 (ver.di 2019b, 78).

As a consequence of the fragmentation in hospital ownership, there is also some fragmentation in the collective actors on the employer's side. Public hospitals as employers at the municipal level are organized in the Vereinigung Kommunaler Arbeitgeberverbände (VKA, Association of Local Government Employers). The Tarifgemeinschaft deutscher Länder (TdL, Bargaining Union of the Federal States) represents university clinics of German states as employers. The Bundesverband Deutscher Privatkliniken (BDPK, Federal Association of Private Clinics) covers private hospital employers. The only private not-for-profit hospital employers' associations are the Verband Kirchlich-Diakonischer Arbeitgeber (VKDA, Association of Church and Diocese Employers) and the Arbeitgeberverband Arbeiterwohlfahrt (Employers Association Workers' Welfare) (Krämer 2011). Both private and public hospital owners are organized as an interest group in the German Hospital Federation (Deutsche Krankenhausgesellschaft, DKG) (DKG 2017).

The structure of collective bargaining in the German hospital sector is highly fragmented, not solely due to the fragmentation in hospital employer associations but also in a three-fold way. Pay, terms, and conditions do not only differ according to (a) hospital ownership but also for (b) different occupational groups and (c) the core and peripheral workforce. Outsourced hospital support services are usually not part of public sector collective agreements (Schulten and Böhlke 2009). In fact, only 10 to 20 per cent of the publicly owned support service subsidiaries are parties to collective agreements. Coverage by an alternative collective agreement is particularly unfavorable for support services workers since the differences to the public sector agreements are highest in the lower wage brackets (Glassner, Pernicka, and Dittmar 2015, 41 f.).

Collective bargaining in the *public* hospitals is still relatively centralized and collective bargaining coverage is high. Most hospital employees are either covered by public sector collective agreements (38.6 per cent by agreements with

VKA, 21.9 per cent by the agreement with the TdL) or agreements with not-for-profit employer organizations (26.3 per cent). Only 1.5 per cent of staff in private hospitals is covered by a collective agreement (Blum, Offermanns, and Perner 2007, 60 ff.).

In the English healthcare sector, employment relations are marked by a typically highly fragmented trade union landscape, but, in contrast to the liberal market economy type of employment relations, also by untypically centralized collective bargaining and an above-average trade union density.

In accordance with the Varieties of Capitalism (VoC) typology, the English trade union landscape is highly fragmented. The main trade unions in the NHS are the general unions UNISON, Unite, and GMB. UNISON, the public services union, covers about 392,000 members in the healthcare services group, which corresponds to 32 per cent of their total membership (UNISON 2017c, 52), out of which about 225,000 are nurses (Prosser 2011). Unite has 100,000 members in the health sector. GMB has 110,000 members in the health sector, of which 85,000 are nurses (Prosser 2011). Similar to ver.di, UNISON is also struggling with declining membership. As such, the number of full members of UNISON dropped from 1.25m in 2014 to 1.22m in 2016 (UNISON 2016, 8, 2017c, 7). 61 per cent of all delegates at the UNISON National Conference in 2016 were female and 28 per cent were working part-time; only 3 per cent were under the age of 27 (UNISON 2017c, 59). Figures specifically on the development of UNISON membership in the NHS were not available. The overall trade union density in the NHS is at a high level of an estimated 58 per cent (Pond 2006; Grimshaw et al. 2007). Members of UNISON pay considerably lower fees than ver.di members. They only pay approximately 0.008 per cent of their annual income to UNISON (UNISON 2017b). The union has a yearly gross income of about £210m from all its units. This is comparable to Unite and about three to four times higher than the budgets of the GMB and Royal College of Nursing (RCN) (Certification Officer 2017, 60). In comparison to ver.di, UNISON is equipped with lower personnel resources. The union employs 1,200 staff throughout the UK (UNISON 2017a), thus working with 0.97 staff per 1,000 members as compared to 1.5 staff per 1,000 ver.di members. However, since trade union membership in the NHS is well above the national average, it can be assumed that UNISON is better equipped with staff here than in its other sectors. Since trade union density in the NHS significantly exceeds the density in the German hospital sector, financial and personnel resources might be more comparable than the calculated average numbers suggest.

In addition to trade unions, there are also two professional associations active in the British hospital sector, the British Medical Association (BMA) for physicians, and the RCN, which covers nurses and assistant nurses. The BMA has about 160,000 members (2017), with an upward tendency (British Medical Association 2017), the RCN has about 420,000 members (Glassner, Pernicka, and Dittmar 2015, 56). The BMA and the RCN are technically trade unions as well. In contrast to the other unions in the sector, they focus more on occupational politics. The BMA went on strike for the first time in 2016 with their junior doctors (Donelly 2016). The RCN considered drawing on their right to strike since 2017 and acted upon it for the first time in December 2019 (RCN 2020).

Collective bargaining in the NHS is in turn untypically centralized due to the vast domination of the NHS in the healthcare sector. The employers' side in the NHS is represented by the NHS employers. All employees employed by the NHS are covered by collective bargaining. However, there is of course a great number of employers in the contracted-out areas. In the private part of the sector, an estimated 40 per cent of employees are covered by collective agreements (Prosser 2011).

1.3.2 General structure of employment in the sector

As shown above, the budget of the German hospital sector makes up 11.7 per cent of GDP (2019) (OECD 2020c). About 1.25m workers were employed in the hospital sector in 2018. This number of employees, however, only adds up to 910,366 full-time equivalents, indicating a high share of part-time employment in this sector. Physicians represented 164,636 full-time equivalents, nurses 331,370 (Statistisches Bundesamt 2020b). Across the EU, about 80 per cent of workers in the health and care sector are women (2005) (Pillinger 2010, 8). Among the caring and nursing personnel, 82 per cent are registered nurses (Aiken et al. 2013, 148). The median gross monthly salary of hospital nurses working full-time amounted to €3,547 in 2019, which is slightly below the German median (Bundesagentur für Arbeit 2019). However, given the high professional, physical, and psychological requirements, as well as the responsibility connected to the nursing profession, the salary is considered as not adequate (Klammer, Klenner, and Lillemeier 2018). Staff shortages in the German hospital sector are increasing. In this way, on average, there were only 39 nurses available nationwide in 2019 compared to 100 registered jobs for nurses in German hospitals (Bundesagentur für Arbeit 2020).

The budget of the NHS makes up 9.8 per cent of British GDP (OECD 2017). A total of 4.1m people are employed in the health and social care sector in the United Kingdom (OECD 2017). 1.5m people are working in the NHS. The NHS England is the largest part of the system, employing 1.2m workers. Of these, 150,273 are hospital doctors, 40,584 are GPs working in practices, 314,966 are nurses and health visitors, 18,862 are ambulance staff, and 111,127 are hospital and community health service (HCHS) medical and dental staff (NHS 2017). 79 per cent of workers in health and social care are female (Pillinger 2010, 40). There is also a large share of hospital employees working part time in the UK. However, this share is decreasing. Part-time work is most prevalent among the nursing workforce. In 2013, 28 per cent of nurses and 35 per cent of nursing auxiliaries and assistants worked part time. These figures are higher in the female nursing workforce, with 40 per cent of female nurses and 40 per cent of nursing auxiliaries and assistants working part time in 2013 (RCN 2014, 8). 28 per cent of registered nurses in England hold a bachelor's degree (Aiken et al. 2013, 145). Wages for nurses and healthcare assistants are well below the national median wage (Pillinger 2010, 39) and have stagnated between 2003 and 2013. NHS pay settlements have not risen above the consumer price index inflation level since 2009. This is in line with the overall low wage growth across the UK economy since the 2008 recession. There is a gender pay gap of 21 per cent in the wider UK economy. Female nurses are still earning 6 per cent less than their male counterparts (RCN 2014, 29 ff.). The relatively small gender pay gap can be attributed to the Agenda for Change pay system, which stipulated job evaluation and a new pay structure with detailed job descriptions. This resulted in overall pay increases, especially in female dominated work (Pillinger 2010, 43).

In contrast to Germany, there is a high and growing share of healthcare assistants in England (RCN 2014). Only 57 per cent of caregivers are professional nurses in England, compared to 82 per cent in Germany (Aiken et al. 2013, 148). Out of all nursing and caring professionals in Great Britain, 35 per cent are nursing professionals and 55 per cent are healthcare assistants (2014) (Eurostat 2016a).

Labor shortages in the UK are so severe that hospital administrators go on expensive recruitment drives, in a bid to hire nursing staff from Europe and non-practising nurses from the UK, or need to use agency staff (RCN 2014, 2 f.).

1.3.3 Trade union responses to marketization and privatization

1.3.3.1 General challenges for trade unions in the hospital sector

Unions face a range of general challenges in the healthcare sector. The main challenges are: (1) a reluctance to strike, stemming from the professional ethos of healthcare employees, the traditional professionalism, and a high share of, supposedly "hard to organize", women in the sector, (2) high fluctuation of employees due to poor working conditions and low pay, and (3) a pragmatic and piecemeal character of reforms.

1   The first obstacle to mobilizing workers in the health sector is their special professional ethos. Especially strike activities are considered as ethically objectionable since they supposedly put patients at risk (Chadwick and Thompson 2000). Some authors argue that a "politicization of caring" (Briskin 2012, 290 f.) or "resistance" framing (Wolf 2015) of this ethos, which draws a connection between striking for better working conditions and improved care quality, can influence the mobilization of nurses positively. This will be examined in more detail in Chapter 6.

Furthermore, there is a tradition of professionalism (Gordon 2009), which entails a focus on providing nurses with educational opportunities and lobbying politicians with research reports, as well as a strict no-strike policy (Jennings and Western 1997). Militancy, i.e. strikes, is a possible strategy in the health sector as well (Briskin 2012). However, this strategy may be problematic if it contradicts professional norms. The potential negative effect of increasing mortality rates through nurses strikes (Gruber and

Kleiner 2012) feeds into nurses' aversion to using strikes. To avoid these problems with professionalism and militancy, US nurse unions have developed a "craft-professional hybrid model" (Ash, Seago, and Spetz 2014, 396) that combines the regulation of patient care through collective bargaining agreements, as well as through public and legislative campaigns. The most prominent example is the minimum staffing levels achieved by the California Nurses Association 1999 (Clark and Clark 2006). In Germany, ver.di developed a new strike policy that secured patient safety during strikes to resolve this dilemma and connected the demand for better working conditions to improving the quality of care (see Chapter 6) In general, framing improved working conditions as a prerequisite for being able to provide satisfactory patient care seems to be suitable to mobilize nurses for industrial action (Reich 2012). In this way, Briskin (2012) has shown this for nurses' strikes in Japan and several European and Anglo-American countries how the dedication to caring and its politicization can encourage rather than dissuade nurses to go on strike.

A third factor contributing to a reluctance to strike is the alleged reluctance of women to strike. Recently, there has been a discussion in the Anglo-American literature on the "feminization "of strikes, i.e., an increasing share of strike activities carried out by women (Briskin 2012). This trend can be attributed to a growing share of female employment and tertiarization or, in other words, the shift of jobs from the manufacturing to the service sector, in which traditionally more women can be found (Dribbusch 2011). The claim that women are "hard to organize" was recently disputed in a variety of studies in the German social and healthcare services (Artus et al. 2017) and by Artus and Pflüger (2017) in their study of the German and Chinese service sector. The authors regard the German social and educational services strikes in 2015 as evidence for the general potential to mobilize women to strike and for actual increasing female strike participation. More than 90 per cent of participants in the 2015 strike were women. However, the strikes were led exclusively by male ver.di officers. In the same way, posts in arbitration were filled by men only.[8] Nevertheless, the authors found that the "collective self-confidence" grew among educators, both female and male, which was also shown by the rejection of the arbitration settlement.

2   Marketization and privatization have a strong effect on working conditions of healthcare workers (Marrs 2007, 4 f.; Greer 2008). A high fluctuation in the workforce due to deteriorating working conditions mainly through work intensification remains another challenge for unions in the healthcare sector. In a study among selected European countries between 11 per cent (Netherlands) and up to 56 per cent (Greece) of nurses reported being dissatisfied with their job. Another 19 per cent (Netherlands) to 49 per cent (Finland and Greece) of nurses intended to leave their current job within one year (Aiken et al. 2013, 147). Accordingly, fluctuation among nurses can be assumed to be just as high, which reduces continuity of trade union activities at the hospital level and further complicates trade unionism in this sector.

3   Last, but not least, the character of marketization reforms and related endeavours can pose a special challenge to unions. Incremental and pragmatically justified reforms or technical policy issues are more difficult to oppose than a single profound and ideologically justified reform (Doellgast and Greer 2007; Givan and Bach 2007). Subsequently, reforms can be hardly politicized at all (Foster and Scott 1998) or salient (Culpepper 2010). This can be observed with the different forms of privatization and marketization. Corporatization and support services outsourcing appear as "lighter" forms of marketization, whereas privatization, outsourcing of medical services, and understaffing are highly politicized. The specific challenges unions are facing with respect to the different forms of marketization and privatization will be discussed in more detail in the corresponding empirical chapters. The next section will portray the main trade union responses to marketization on the national level.

1.3.3.2 National-level trade union responses to marketization

Trade unions have responded to the marketization trends described above in various ways. However, relatively little has been done to stop or influence reforms on the national level early on.

Ver.di did not manage to prevent national-level reforms in the hospital sector such as the introduction of the DRGs in 2003, but managed to exert some influence on healthcare financing. Its "Gesundheitskampagne" was intended to influence the 2002 bill that created DRGs, but was not effective, which can also be attributed to the fact that the union had newly been founded and the five original unions still had to learn how to run a campaign together (ver.di 2003). Even though ver.di did not have much influence on the design of markets in the 2002 reforms, it managed to gain a €3.5bn euro hospital funding increase in 2009 by working in a broad healthcare coalition and mobilizing 130,000 workers in its Remove the Cap campaign ("Der Deckel muss weg") (Greer, Schulten, and Böhlke 2013, 225 f.) (ver.di Infodienst Krankenhäuser 10/2008). Through the Release the Pressure campaign ("Der Druck muss raus") and years of action, ver.di has brought the issue of understaffing to the attention of federal lawmakers. Ver.di succeeded at pushing for the adoption of a law that obliges hospital associations and health insurance funds to draft mandatory minimum staffing levels for "care-sensitive" areas by the beginning of 2019 (Bundesministerium für Gesundheit 2017). These minimum staffing levels have been widely criticized as being insufficient. They are not suitable to guarantee high care quality and good working conditions but merely aim at preventing patient damage. In the meantime, ver.di was also active on the local level and negotiated nearly 20 agreements since 2015 with mainly university hospitals that stipulate safe staffing levels allowing for high care quality (ver.di 2019a). The pathway to the first agreement of this kind at Charité Berlin will be described in Chapter 6. In 2020, an unusual alliance of ver.di, the German Hospital Federation, and the German Nursing Council demanded replacing the minimum staffing levels of 2019 with an updated version of the needs-oriented staffing levels ("Pflegepersonalregelung, PPR 2.0") that they had tested in 50 hospitals (DKG 2020; ver.di 2020).

For the English unions, it was possible to benefit from national legal regulations. These mostly concerned, first, the British implementation of the European directive regarding outsourcing workers and, second, pay increases arising from the new pay structure contained in the Agenda for Change. Great significance can be attributed to the regulations governing the transfer of workers in outsourcing processes, the TUPE, and two-tier code. However, these were withdrawn respectively loosened in 2014 and can be easily circumvented (see Section 1.2.1.2). To halt the compulsory outsourcing of ancillary staff as part of PFI projects, the option of "Retention of Employment" was introduced. It allows NHS employers to retain nonsupervisory staff. Only supervisory, estate, and maintenance staff need to be outsourced. This policy was a response to union campaigns to protect NHS workers' generous public sector pensions that are not covered by the TUPE legislation (Grimshaw 2009).

Under New Labour, unions were also more successful at concluding other agreements in the sector. In 2004, after unrest due to higher remuneration of ancillary workers in comparison to qualified nurses, and four years of negotiation, the Labour government agreed with trade unions on the Agenda for Change. Implemented in 2006, the Agenda for Change reorganized staff grades and linked pay to performance through a Knowledge and Skills Framework which determined skill levels necessary for pay progression (Bach and Kessler 2012, 48, 64 ff.). Eventually, as there were no new positions created, the performance-related career advancement did not have a strong impact. At the same time, the Agenda for Change increased pay significantly, especially for low-wage workers, but also for nurses, due to UNISON's strong campaign on this issue (Grimshaw 2009, 452 ff.; Bach and Kessler 2012, 60). In 2014, the British unions were also successful at achieving staff increases as a result of the care quality scandals and their campaign for safe staffing levels (RCN 2014, 15).

There are few empirical studies dealing with *local-level* trade union responses to hospital sector marketization and privatization in Germany and Britain. Most research deals with outsourcing of support services in the British public sector, but there is little research on corporatization, privatization, and understaffing in the hospital sector in general. The main challenges for unions in the specific marketization processes will be portrayed in the according empirical chapters.

1.4 Research design and methods

The book aims to contribute a structured focused comparison of trade union responses to health sector marketization and privatization and its understaffing effects in Germany and England. To this end, the following questions are posed: How do trade unions respond to marketization processes? Why do they choose which strategy? Why do unions in different countries choose the same strategies? And, with respect to Chapters 5 and 6, what are the determinants of successful strategies? These questions will be answered following a most-different systems research design containing 19 case studies.

1.4.1 Research design

The empirical analysis presented in this book consists of 19 case studies presented in four empirical chapters. Cases in these chapters are defined as trade union strategies designed to combat marketization or contain its effects. All case studies are theory-centered (Rohlfing 2012, 1–22), setup as structured focused and contextualized comparisons (Geddes 2003, 137), and embedded in most-different systems (Przeworski and Teune 1970). They are based on documents from trade union magazines and other media outlets, as well as interviews mainly with trade unionists. The material was analysed using qualitative content analysis (Mayring 2008) and, where the material was dense enough, elements of process tracing (Beach and Pedersen 2013).

The most-different systems design is marked by a comparable outcome of the cases that is least likely to occur due to the different systems the outcome was produced in. Systemic factors are not given any special place among the possible predictors of behavior (Przeworski and Teune 1970, 34 f.). The comparison is contextualized, taking into account that phenomena in two different contexts can play out differently and yet be *analytically equivalent* (Locke and Thelen 1995, 11). This means that though the concrete manifestations of dynamics may be different, they operate as functional equivalents and have the same consequences. In this book, conflicts stemming from different forms of marketization in two countries that are least likely to produce similar trade union strategies considering their macro-institutional settings – Germany and Great Britain – are compared to gain insights into sub-national and agency factors that determine trade union strategies and, in Chapters 5 and 6, also their outcome. Chapter 6 also features a US American case study on the struggle for mandatory staffing levels due to its striking parallels to the German case.

The selected cases differ with respect to their macro-institutional contexts. The two *healthcare systems* are clearly distinct from one another. The German healthcare system can be characterized as of "social insurance" or Bismarckian type, Great Britain has a state-dominated "NHS" type healthcare system (for more details on the healthcare systems, see Section 1.2). Comparative *employment relations* theory treats Germany and Great Britain as coordinated and liberal market economy types respectively. This framework generally does not fit the experience of public sector unions (Bach and Bordogna 2011). Characteristics of the German and English *healthcare sector employment relations* differ from these ideal types in certain respects. The German healthcare sector is marked by an unusually fragmented collective bargaining landscape along the lines of hospital ownership, professions, as well as core and periphery workers. However, collective bargaining in the *public* hospitals is relatively centralized. In turn, collective bargaining in the NHS is untypically centralized. Fitting the VoC typology, the trade union landscape is highly fragmented in England, while it is

Table 1.6 Research design overview

	Healthcare system	Employment relations	Marketization Processes (main independent variable)	Outcome (dependent variable: strategic union choice)
Germany	Bismarckian, social security type	Coordinated	Marketization processes creating political opportunity structures	Comparable strategies deployed as a response to different forms of marketization
England	Beveridge, NHS type	Liberal		

Source: Böhm et al. (2013), Rothgang et al. (2005), Hall and Soskice (2001), Bambra (2005), Bach and Bordogna (2011), own presentation.

rather centralized in Germany. Trade union density in Germany is slightly above the national average, whereas it is markedly higher in England. In contrast to England, also in the public healthcare sector, German unions possess the usual extensive co-determination rights (Krämer 2011; Frosser 2011; Glassner, Pernicka, and Dittmar 2015). Although the characteristics of employment relations in the healthcare sectors are not in line with the VoC characteristics and the national average, they reflect the general national features and can clearly be regarded as distinct in the two countries.

Based on this national-level setting, one would expect trade unions to be confronted with different challenges and, accordingly, to pursue different goals and choose different strategies. However, the case studies show that marketization creates similar opportunity structures, i.e., similar pressures and opportunities to act, which not only put trade unions in a defensive position but can also be used by the unions to their benefit and produce certain comparable strategies – which is the outcome of interest. Trade unions pursued the same goals of resisting marketization or containing its work intensification effects by using similar strategies depending on the form of marketization. This is attributed to similar opportunity structures and an effective use of resources, depending on the unions' capabilities (see Table 1.6).

This book encompasses 19 case studies in total. These are composed of 7 in-depth case studies (Chapter 3, 4, and 6). Another 12 shorter case studies are presented in Chapter 5. This medium-N sample allows the analysis at the cross-case level, between the two countries and the different forms of marketization. In the following section, the selection of cases will be described.

1.4.2 Case selection

The selection of the cases is mostly guided by the theoretical framework. It should be relevant for the research question and, more specifically, suitable to study the following proposition:

Table 1.7 Logic of case selection

	Formal privatization (corporatization)	Functional privatization (outsourcing)	Material privatization	Staffing levels
Germany	1 case	1 case	6 cases	1 case
England	1 case	1 case	6 cases	1 case
USA	-	-	-	1 case

Source: Own presentation.

Marketization in the two countries follows the same directionality and creates similar opportunity structures, i.e., similar problems and pressures to act. These will provoke comparable trade union action that depends on the trade union's local resources and capabilities.

Appropriate cases were identified and sampled at the country level and with respect to the three main marketization forms (Bryman 2012, 417). The choice of countries was to maximize variation between national institutional structures. Germany and England are least similar with respect to their welfare state, employment relations and healthcare system as outlined in the previous section. Furthermore, cases were selected to account for the variation in the forms of marketization around which conflicts on the hospital level can evolve. The cases cover the most relevant forms of marketization – corporatization, outsourcing, and material privatization – which often occur in combination and/or build on one another. These are complemented by another type of conflict evoked by marketization, namely the pursuit of mandatory staffing levels (see Table 1.7). Studying conflicts arising from all relevant forms of marketization allows examining how far strategies designed to combat marketization vary with respect to the intensity of marketization, the interest of the public in the specific matter, its effects on the whole workforce and on different parts of it. Also, the unions' rationale, the relevance they attribute to the conflict, as well as their aim vary with the form of marketization. Consequently, a union might strive for the *prevention* of privatization in one case, while pursuing efforts aimed at containment in the case of support service outsourcing, and adapt their strategic choice accordingly. The type of marketization might also affect the public support the union can expect and the possibilities to enter coalitions with civil society actors. The comparison allows assessing whether the rationale of strategic union choices and chances for success change from one form of marketization to another.

Furthermore, the healthcare sector was chosen because of the various and profound marketization processes (see Section 1.2) and the recent dynamic development of trade unionism in this sector among nurses. Activism of nurses is regarded as unlikely due to the nurses' professional ethic (Chadwick and Thompson 2000). The recent increased use of strikes in this sector, in particular those including nurses, can therefore be regarded as least likely cases (Gerring 2007, 118 f.) that add "probative value" (Rohlfing 2012, 16). Moreover, the choice of the hospital sector is motivated by the variety of heterogeneous professions, which poses a special challenge for trade unions. Furthermore, organizing nurses is interesting not only because of their professional ethic but also because their profession is characterized by a high share of supposedly hard-to-organize women, part-time work and pay (see Section 1.3.2). Trade unions are, thus, faced with a particular and challenging situation in this sector that is worth studying.

The case studies focus on the main trade unions in the two health sectors, UNISON and ver.di. The choice of these unions is motivated by their size in the sector, as well as the variety of professions they cover in the health sector (sectors see Section 1.3.1).

Moreover, the selected conflicts had to be of relevance and of a certain salience. This criterion was important to assure sufficient coverage in trade union magazines and media, as well as general trade union activity in the conflict. Furthermore, cases were supposed to be typical (Bryman 2012, 419) to allow for more general conclusions about trade union strategies in the sectors of the two countries. To reduce possible sources of variation between the matched cases stemming from location (rural/urban) and size of the hospitals (number of beds, employees, and annual turnover), these factors were kept stable. Additionally, regarding the German cases, only conflicts in hospitals with public ownership were studied to fit better with the English cases and, again, to reduce variation among the German cases stemming from this factor. Lastly, to match the most-different systems design, the matched cases had to be comparable in their outcomes, i.e., the trade unions' strategic choices.

The cases were identified mainly through document analysis. For England, additional interviews with national and regional trade unionists were conducted, since the analysed documents were not as rich in information about marketization conflicts as the German ones. The selection of cases did not aim at composing a representative sample of trade union responses to health sector marketization that would allow for generalization (Bryman 2012, 422). Instead, it aims at providing a comprehensive overview with a focus on the facets of marketization and an investigation of determinants of (successful) trade union strategies. For an overview of the characteristics of the cases studied, see Tables 1.8 and 1.9. A short summary of the cases studied will be given at the end of this chapter in Section 1.5.

The cases studied show differing temporalities in two respects. First, the formal privatization case studies took place earlier than most of the case studies of other forms of marketization. As described earlier in this chapter, this can be attributed to the different forms of marketization building on one another. Furthermore, formal privatization became less contested and was, thus, less reported over time. Second, cases of material privatization in Germany and cases of medical services commissioning took place at different times as well. In Germany, material privatization was possible at any point in time, since the private provision of healthcare is a characteristic of the Bismarckian healthcare system. Prompted by reunification and the introduction of the DRGs, there were two privatization waves, one in the 1990s and another one in the mid-2000s.

Table 1.8 Case studies of union strategies regarding three types of marketization in Germany and England

Marketization type	Germany				England			
	Year	Case characteristics	Strategies	Outcome	Year	Case characteristics	Strategies	Outcome
Corporatization Cases	2001	Large metropolitan hospital, relatively early case; typical case; main actors: local trade unionists and workplace representatives	Partnership, proactively interpreted	Transformation with significant influence by the union	2004	Large metropolitan hospital, relatively early case; typical case; main actors: local trade unionists, and workplace representatives	Partnership	Transformation without significant union involvement
Outsourcing Cases	2015–2017	Large metropolitan hospital; relatively late but typical case; main actors: local trade unionists and workplace representatives	Partnership and organizing	Outsourcing with extended effects bargaining, ongoing reversal efforts	2015–2017	Large metropolitan hospital, relatively late, and particularly 'successful' case as rated by UNISON; main actors: local trade unionists and workplace representatives, supported at the national level	Partnership and organizing	Outsourcing with necessary continuous effects bargaining; however, no membership losses as usual

(Continued)

Table 1.8 (Continued)

Marketization type	Germany				England			
	Year	Case characteristics	Strategies	Outcome	Year	Case characteristics	Strategies	Outcome
Privatization cases	2004–2010	All cases of large hospital privatization (hospitals with more than 900 beds) (6 cases); main actors: local trade unionists and workplace representatives	Mostly social movement unionism	Privatization usually not avoided, despite vigorous campaigns	2014–2015	All cases of large medical services commissioning exercises (above £60m value) (6 cases); main actors: local trade unionists, workplace representatives, and grassroots campaigners	Social movement unionism	Privatization usually avoided, but campaigns often led by grassroots or competing union (Unite)

Source: Own presentation.

Table 1.9 Case studies of union strategies for staffing levels in Germany, England and the USA

| Marketization type | Germany | | | | England | | | | USA | | | |
	Year	Case characteristics	Strategies	Outcome	Year	Case characteristics	Main strategy	Outcome	Year	Case characteristics	Strategies	Outcome
Understaffing cases	2013–2016	Large metropolitan hospital; first outstanding, but exemplary case in Germany and accompanying national campaign	Social movement unionism and organizing	In-house collective agreement stipulating mandatory staffing levels	2013	Large metropolitan hospitals; pilot pro-jects and accompanying national campaign	Partner-ship and lobbying	Topic of mandatory staffing levels on the political agenda	2012–2016	Large metropolitan hospitals; first outstanding case in New York State and accompanying state-wide campaign	Social movement unionism and organizing	Multi-employer collective agreement stipulating mandatory staffing levels

Source: Own presentation.

Therefore, the time period under consideration stretches from 1996 to 2010. In Britain, commissioning of medical services was only enabled through the HSCA in 2012, and therefore cases of large-scale medical services commissioning could only be found from 2014 onwards. Chapter 6 features a second comparison of the German case with an US American case. This is motivated by its striking parallels to the German case with respect to the trade unions' resources, capabilities, and strategic choices. The US American healthcare and employment relations systems can be regarded as most different from the German as well.

1.4.3 Data and methods

This section explains how data was collected and analyzed. All case studies are based on two types of qualitative data.

1.4.3.1 Documents

The first type of source were articles of regularly published trade union magazines from 2001 to 2016, as well as selected social media and newspaper articles. For Germany, I analyzed the quarterly publication of the United Services Union (ver.di). Since December 2001, the hospital sector unit of ver.di issues its own magazine named "Infodienst Krankenhäuser". All articles in ver.di's "Infodienst Krankenhäuser" between 12/2001 and 4/2016 were taken into account. All issues together amounted to roughly 3,835 pages. I selected 422 articles from 65 issues. Quotes from this publication will be marked as "IK" followed by the month and year of the quoted issue.

For England, I analyzed the UNISON InFocus magazine, a journal for UNISON activists that, in contrast to the "Infodienst Krankenhäuser", is not sector-specific. It has been published since 1995. I studied all 177 issues of the journal from 01/2002 until 02/2015. All issues together amounted to about 4,677 pages in total (864 pages of UNISONFocus 2002–2004 and 3,813 pages of UNISON InFocus 2004–2015). From the 177 studied issues, I selected 348 articles.

All journal articles dealing with conflicts about marketization or its effects in the hospital sectors were selected, summarized, and analyzed using a deductively derived category system to structure the material (Mayring 2008, 92 ff.). Additional documents from union magazines, newspapers, governance websites, and social media were not coded, but merely used as sources.

1.4.3.2 Interviews

Based on the information gained through the document analysis and additional interviews with English trade unionists, comparable cases were selected for further investigation by means of interviews in the second phase. The in-depth analyses are based on 35 original interviews with trade unionists, activists, management and a local politician, conducted between September 2015 and March 2016. Chapters 5 and 6 are based on 88 interviews (2003–2007 and 2015–2016), respectively, 14 more interviews (2015–2017).[9] Quotes from interviews will be marked as "IP", followed by the corresponding interview number (and if available page or section).

The method of expert interviewing (Bogner, Littig, and Menz 2009) was suitable, since it allowed me to gather detailed information on the conflict processes and to understand the actors' motives for action. The interview was deployed to systematically reconstruct the process of the conflict, as well as to study the theoretical assumptions (Bogner and Menz 2009; Littig 2011). In combination with the information from document analysis, it allowed for the reconstruction of the process to a certain degree (Rohlfing 2012, 150–167; Beach and Pedersen 2013).

1.5 Structure of the book

In this introductory chapter, I have given an overview of the different healthcare systems and marketization policies in Germany and England, the structure of the sectors, the effects of marketization on trade unions, and the special challenges they are facing. The research design and methods were briefly laid out.

Building on previous works, I will present an existing theoretical framework that accounts for the transformative effect of social and economic change and will extend it with concepts focusing on the local-level leeway that trade unions can use if they build up and mobilize the corresponding resources and capacities (Chapter 2).

The first three empirical chapters are dedicated to the three most common forms of marketization and the corresponding trade union reactions (Chapters 3, 4, and 5). The fourth empirical chapter will examine the containment of negative effects of marketization for workers through mandatory staffing levels (Chapter 6)

In more detail, Chapter 3 studies two cases of trade union strategies opposing corporatization in large metropolitan hospitals that took place in the early 2000s. The cases represent two relatively early, but typical cases. Furthermore, at least for Germany, there have been few recent cases of corporatization that were reported in the union media due to their low politicization and a desensitization effect. Trade unionists in both cases did not oppose corporatization, and therefore used a partnership strategy, though with differing outcomes. While trade unionists in England were informed about, but did not have a significant influence during the transformation process, German trade unionists pursued a more proactive partnership approach, successfully making suggestions to combine the corporatization with a merger to make the municipal hospitals more competitive and thus safeguard jobs in the long term.

Chapter 4 studies two relatively late cases of outsourcing of hospital support services in large metropolitan hospitals between 2015 and 2017. The German case can be regarded as typical. The English case was evaluated as particularly successful. It was chosen since the English union usually remained quiescent during more recent outsourcing processes, and there were only few outsourcing cases mentioned in the analyzed trade union magazine, predominantly with little trade union activity. In both cases studied, most of the union representatives did not oppose the outsourcing and therefore, pursued a partnership approach to bargain over effects of the outsourcing. At the same time, both unions made efforts to retain their members who were affected by the outsourcing and to organize new workers in the outsourced services. In both cases, negative effects, such as the deterioration of wages, terms, and conditions, were widely prevented. However, it necessitated continued efforts of the English union to fight off later deteriorations. The German union also sustained their activities after the outsourcing, proactively pushing for the same wages, terms and conditions of new workers and insourcing outsourced services.

Chapter 5 studies all cases of large-scale privatization of hospitals with more than 900 beds in Germany from 2004 to 2010 (6 cases), and all cases of large-scale medical service commissions of more than £60m value in England from 2014 to 2015 (6 cases). All cases of privatization were strongly opposed by unions and, in England, also by grassroots campaign groups. Anti-privatization campaigns in both countries usually drew on social movement unionism and were widely supported by the public. Nevertheless, campaigns in Germany usually did not prevent hospital privatization while in England they usually succeeded in avoiding the commissioning of medical services to a private sector provider.

Chapter 6 studies three cases of campaigns for mandatory staffing levels on both the national level and the workplace level in Germany, England, as well as in the USA, namely the State of New York. The additional comparison with a US American case is motivated by its striking parallels to the German case with respect to the trade unions' resources, capacities, and strategic choices. Both cases took place between 2012–2013 and 2016, and represent first outstandingly successful attempts to achieve mandatory staffing levels laid down in collective agreements, deploying a combination of social movement unionism, and organizing. Unions in England have also been active in promoting staffing levels since 2012. In contrast to the aforementioned cases, they pursued a partnership approach at the shop level. At the national level, they connected with a network of allies, but did not use it in terms of social movement unionism. These strategies have so far not been successful.

The results of the four empirical chapters are synthesized in the final chapter that identifies determinants of (successful) trade union strategies. The findings highlight the relevance of sector-specific marketization and the corresponding political opportunities that need to be recognized by unions. Marketization processes appear to overlay traditional employment relations types and provide leeway to local-level trade unionism which, in turn, then depends on local-level power resources and capabilities. The studies have also shown the limits of strategies, especially of the partnership strategy, when the necessary resources and capabilities are missing. The results hint at the importance of strategies that match local-level resources and capabilities, and the possibility to build them. The findings also point to a link between intensifying marketization and increasing salience of the issue. Since healthcare is a topic of general public interest, promoting marketization can increase the value of societal power. In this context, strategies based on social movement unionism appear a logical choice for unions, especially in anti-privatization campaigns and campaigns to improve staffing levels. On the basis of the empirical findings, a refined theoretical model of trade union strategic choice in times of marketization will be suggested, drawing conclusions for trade unionism practice in the marketized health sector (Chapter 7).

Notes

1. Furthermore, the situation in Scotland and Wales differs from England as devolution in 1999 has led to a reversal of marketization processes and would therefore not be comparable (Leys and Player 2011, 150–153).
2. Department of Health and Social Security Circular HC (83) 18 – Health Services Management: Competitive Tendering in the Provision of Domestic, Catering and Laundry Services.
3. Since 1999, the Fair Deal for Staff Pensions ruled that contractors had to offer comparable occupational pension schemes. It was reformed in 2013 and, since then, gives transferred staff access to the public service pension scheme (UNISON 2014).
4. There are certain possibilities for employers to completely circumvent the application of the TUPE regulations. This is the case for "framework agreements" about services that will be delivered on demand or in case of the "Any Qualified Provider" policy of the NHS that allows patients to choose from a list of providers of healthcare services (UNISON 2014, 16).
5. Information on the extent of contracted out support services is not held centrally, and thus figures on this matter are not available.
6. In this way, performance also depends on how ambitious the staffing levels that hospitals set for themselves are.
7. Several more unions are also active in the German hospital sector, such as the Beamtenbund und Tarifunion (dbb), the Christlicher Gewerkschaftsbund (CGB), Verband kirchlicher Mitarbeiter und Mitarbeiterinnen (VKM), or Gewerkschaft Kirche und Diakonie (GKD). Their total membership can be considered markedly lower than those of ver.di and the Marburger Bund in this sector (Krämer 2011) and will therefore not be treated in more detail.
8. However, the authors noted, this strike yielded greater gains on a symbolic level, i.e., for the recognition of the profession as equal to typically male jobs that require similarly high qualifications than on the financial level. This was attributed to a lack of structural power and a weak economic effect of strikes in the social and educational services (Artus and Pflüger 2017).
9. Interviews and analyses of these additional interviews were generously provided by Ian Greer, Nick Krachler, and Geneviève Coderre-LaPalme.

References

ACAS. 2014. 2014 Changes to TUPE. http://www.acas.org.uk/media/pdf/t/r/9908-2901767-TSO-ACAS-TUPE_is_changing-ACCESSIBLE.pdf.

Aiken, Linda H., Douglas M. Sloane, Jeannie P. Cimiotti, Sean P. Clarke, Linda Flynn, Jean Ann Seago, Joanne Spetz, and Herbert L. Smith. 2010. Implications of the California Nurse Staffing Mandate for Other States. *Health Services Research* no. 45 (4):904–921.

Aiken, Linda H., Douglas M. Sloane, Luk Bruyneel, Koen Van den Heede, Peter Griffiths, Reinhard Busse, Marianna Diomidous, Juha Kinnunen, Maria Kózka, Emmanuel Lesaffre, Matthew D. McHugh, M. T. Moreno-Casbas, Anne Marie Rafferty, Rene

Schwendimann, P. Anne Scott, Carol Tishelman, Theo van Achterberg, and Walter Sermeus. 2014. Nurse Staffing and Education and Hospital Mortality in Nine European Countries: A Retrospective Observational Study. *Lancet* no. 383:1824–1830.

Aiken, Linda H., Douglas M. Sloane, Luk Bruyneel, Koen Van den Heede, and Walter Sermeus. 2013. Nurses' Reports of Working Conditions and Hospital Quality of Care in 12 Countries in Europe. *International Journal of Nursing Studies* no. 50 (2):143–153.

Aiken, Linda H., Jeannie P. Cimiotti, Douglas M. Sloane, Herbert L. Smith, Linda Flynn, and Donna F. Neff. 2011. Effects of Nurse Staffing and Nurse Education on Patient Deaths in Hospitals with Different Nurse Work Environments. *Medical Care* no. 49 (12):1047–1053.

André, Christine, and Christoph Hermann. 2009. Privatisation and Marketisation of Health Care Systems in Europe. In *Privatization against the European Social Model. A Critique of European Policies and Proposals for Alternatives*, edited by Marica Frangakis, Christoph Hermann, Jörg Huffschmid and Károly Lóránt, 129–144. Basingstoke: Palgrave Macmillan.

Arora, Sandeepa, Anita Charlesworth, Elaine Kelly, and George Stoye. 2013. *Public Payment and Private Provision: The Changing Landscape of Health Care in the 2000s.* London: Nuffield Trust.

Artus, Ingrid, and Jessica Pflüger. 2017. Streik und Gender in Deutschland und China: Ein explorativer Blick auf aktuelles Streikgeschehen. *Industrielle Beziehungen* no. 2:218–240.

Artus, Ingrid, Peter Birke, Stefan Kerber-Clasen, and Wolfgang Menz. 2017. *Sorge-Kämpfe: Auseinandersetzungen um Arbeit in Sozialen Dienstleistungen.* Hamburg: VSA Verlag.

Ash, Michael, Jean A. Seago, and Joanne Spetz. 2014. What Do Health Care Unions Do?: A Response to Manthous. *Medical Care* no. 52 (5):393–397.

Augurzky, Boris, Rosemarie Gülker, Roman Mennicken, Stefan Felder, Setan Meyer, Jürgen Wasem, Hartmut Gülker, and Nikolaus Siemssen. 2012. Mengenentwicklung und Mengensteuerung stationärer Leistungen: Endbericht. Essen: Rheinisch-Westfälisches Institut für Wirtschaftsforschung (RWI). http://nbn-resolving.de/urn:nbn:de:hbz:061:3-20199.

Augurzky, Boris, Sebastian Krolop, Adam Pilny, Christoph Schmidt, and Christiane Wuckel. 2020. *Krankenhaus Rating Report 2020: Ende einer Ära. Aufbruch ins neue Jahrzehnt.* Heidelberg: medhochzwei.

Augurzky, Boris, Sebastian Krolop, and Christoph M. Schmidt. 2010. Die wirtschaftliche Lage der Krankenhäuser. In *Krankenhaus-Report 2010*, edited by Jürgen Klauber, Max Gareadts and Jörg Friedrich, 13–24. Stuttgart: Schattauer.

Bach, Stephen, and Ian Kessler. 2012. *The Modernisation of the Public Services and Employee Relations: Targeted Change.* Basingstoke: Palgrave Macmillan.

Bach, Stephen, Ian Kessler, and Paul Heron. 2012. Nursing a Grievance? The Role of Healthcare Assistants in a Modernized National Health Service. *Gender, Work and Organization* no. 19 (2):205–224.

Bach, Stephen, and Lorenzo Bordogna. 2011. Varieties of New Public Management or Alternative Models? The Reform of Public Service Employment Relations in Industrialized Democracies. *International Journal of Human Resource Management* no. 22 (11):2349–2366.

Baggott, Rob. 2004. *Health and Health Care in Britain.* 3rd edition. Basingstoke: Macmillan Education.

Bambra, Clare. 2005. Worlds of Welfare and the Health Care Discrepancy. *Social Policy and Society* no. 4 (1):31–41.

Beach, Derek, and Rasmus Brun Pedersen. 2013. *Process-Tracing Methods: Foundations and Guidelines*. Ann Arbor: The University of Michigan Press.

Bishop, Simon, and Justin Waring. 2011. Inconsistency in Health Care Professional Work: Employment in Independent Sector Treatment Centres. *Journal of Health Organisation and Management* no. 25 (3):315–331.

Blum, Karl, Matthias Offermanns, and Patricia Perner. 2007. *Krankenhaus Barometer: Umfrage 2007*. Düsseldorf: Deutsches Krankenhausinstitut e.V.

Blum, Karl, Sabine Löffert, Matthias Offermans, and Petra Steffen. 2013. Krankenhaus Barometer: Umfrage 2013. Düsseldorf: Deutsches Krankenhausinstitut e.V. https://www.dki.de/sites/default/files/downloads/krankenhaus_barometer_2013.pdf.

Blum, Karl, Sabine Löffert, Matthias Offermans, and Petra Steffen. 2015. Krankenhaus-Barometer: Umfrage 2015. Düsseldorf: Deutsches Krankenhausinstitut e.V.

Blum, Karl, Sabine Löffert, Matthias Offermans, and Petra Steffen. 2016. Krankenhaus-Barometer: Umfrage 2016. Düsseldorf: Deutsches Krankenhausinstitut e.V.

Blumenthal, David, Melinda Abrams, and Rachel Nuzum. 2015. The Affordable Care Act at 5 Years. *New England Journal of Medicine* no. 372:2451–2458.

Bogner, Alexander, Beate Littig, and Wolfgang Menz. 2009. *Interviewing Experts*. Basingstoke/New York: Palgrave Macmillan.

Bogner, Alexander, and Wolfgang Menz. 2009. The Theory-Generating Expert Interview: Epistemological Interest, Forms of Knowledge, Interaction. In *Interviewing Experts*, edited by Alexander Bogner, Beate Littig and Wolfgang Menz, 43–80. Basingstoke/New York: Palgrave Macmillan.

Böhlke, Nils, Ian Greer, and Thorsten Schulten. 2011. World Champions in Hospital Privatisation: The Effects of Neoliberal Reform on German Employees and Patients. https://ecommons.cornell.edu/handle/1813/75252.

Böhm, Katharina, Achim Schmid, Ralf Götze, Claudia Landwehr, and Heinz Rothgang. 2013. Five Types of OECD Healthcare Systems: Empirical Results of a Deductive Classification. *Health Policy* no. 113 (3):258–269. http://dx.doi.org/10.1016/j.healthpol.2013.09.003.

Boyle, Seán. 2011. United Kingdom (England): Health System Review. *Health Systems in Transition* no. 13 (1):1–486.

Briskin, Linda. 2012. Resistance, Mobilization and Militancy: Nurses on Strike. *Nursing Inquiry* no. 19 (4):285–296.

British Medical Association. 2017. Membership. https://www.bma.org.uk/membership.

Bryman, Alan. 2012. *Social Research Methods*. Oxford: Oxford University Press.

Bund, Marburger. 2020. Wir sind... https://www.marburger-bund.de/bundesverband/der-marburger-bund/der-verband/ihre-interessenvertretung/wir-sind.

Bundesagentur für Arbeit. 2019. Entgelt für den Beruf: Gesundheits- und Krankenpfleger/in. https://con.arbeitsagentur.de/prod/entgeltatlas/beruf/27355.

Bundesagentur für Arbeit. 2020. Arbeitsmarktsituation im Pflegebereich. https://statistik.arbeitsagentur.de/DE/Statischer-Content/Statistiken/Themen-im-Fokus/Berufe/Generische-Publikationen/Altenpflege.pdf?__blob=publicationFile&v=8.

Bundesministerium für Gesundheit. 2017. Schlussfolgerungen aus den Beratungen der Expertinnen- und Expertenkommission "Pflegepersonal im Krankenhaus". Berlin, 7. März. https://www.bundesgesundheitsministerium.de/fileadmin/Dateien/3_Downloads/P/Pflegekommisison/170307_Abschlusspapier_Pflegekommission.pdf.

Busse, Reinhard, and Annette Riesberg. 2005. *Gesundheitssysteme im Wandel: Deutschland*. Kopenhagen: WHO Regionalbüro für Europa im Auftrag des Europäischen Observatoriums für Gesundheitssysteme und Gesundheitspolitik.

Cabinet Office. 2010a. Principles of Good Employment Practice: A Statement of Principles that Reflect Good Employment Practice for Governmen, Contracting Authorities and Suppliers. https://www.gov.uk/government/uploads/system/uploads/attachment_data/file/62089/principles-good-employment.pdf.

Cabinet Office. 2010b. Two-Tier Code Withdrawn. https://www.gov.uk/government/news/two-tier-code-withdrawn.

Certification Officer. 2017. Annual Report of the Certification Officer 2016-2017. https://www.gov.uk/government/uploads/system/uploads/attachment_data/file/629399/Cert_Off_Ann_Rep_2016-2017.pdf.

Chadwick, Ruth, and Alison Thompson. 2000. Professional Ethics and Labor Disputes: Medicine and Nursing in the United Kingdom. *Cambridge Quarterly of Healthcare Ethics* no. 9:483–497.

Clark, Darlene A., and Paul F. Clark.. 2006. Union Strategies for Improving Patient Care: The Key to Nurse Unionism. *Labor Studies Journal* no. 31 (1):51–70.

Clark, Paul. F, Darlene A. Clark, David V. Day, and Dennis G. Shea. 2001. Healthcare Reform and the Workplace Experience of Nurses: Implications for Patient Care and Union Organizing. *Industrial and Labor Relations Review* no. 55 (133).

Conservative Party. 1983. The Challenge of Our Times. Election Manifesto. https://www.margaretthatcher.org/document/110859.

Cousins, Christine. 1988. The Restructuring of Welfare Work: The Introduction of General Management and the Contracting Out of Ancillary Services in the NHS. *Work, Employment & Society* no. 2:210–228.

Culpepper, Pepper D. 2010. *Quiet Politics and Business Power: Corporate Control in Europe and Japan.* New York: Cambridge University Press.

Cylus, Jonathan, Erica Richardson, Lisa Findley, Marcus Longley, O'Neill Ciaran, and David Steel. 2015. United Kingdom: Health System Review. *Health Systems in Transition* no. 17 (5):1–125.

Davies, Anne C. L. 2013. This Time, It's for Real: The Health and Social Care Act 2012. *The Modern Law Review* no. 76 (3):564–588.

Davies, Steve. 2005. *Hospital Contract Cleaning and Infection Control.* London: UNISON.

Department of Health. 2000. The NHS Plan: A Plan for Investment – A Plan for Reform. http://webarchive.nationalarchives.gov.uk/20130107105354/http://www.dh.gov.uk/prod_consum_dh/groups/dh_digitalassets/@dh/@en/@ps/documents/digitalasset/dh_118522.pdf.

Department of Trade and Industry. 2007. Employment Rights on the Transfer of an Undertaking: A Guide to the 2006 TUPE Regulations for Employees, Employers, and Representatives. http://webarchive.nationalarchives.gov.uk/20070603164510/http://www.dti.gov.uk/files/file20761.pdf.

Deutscher Gewerkschaftsbund. 2020. DGB Mitgliederzahlen 2000-2009, 2010-2019. http://www.dgb.de/uber-uns/dgb-heute/mitgliederzahlen.

Deutsches Krankenhausinstitut. 2005. Krankenhausbarometer Umfrage 2005. http://www.dkgev.de/media/file/1856.Umfrage_2005.pdf.

DKG. 2017. Mission and Objectives. http://www.dkgev.de/dkg.php/cat/257/aid/10696.

DKG. 2020. Ein Pflegepersonabedarfsbemessungsinstrument. https://www.dkgev.de/themen/personal-weiterbildung/ppr-20/.

Doellgast, Virginia, and Ian Greer. 2007. Vertical Disintegration and the Disorganization of German Industrial Relations. *British Journal of Industrial Relations* no. 45 (1):55–76.

Donelly, Laura. 2016. As Junior Doctors Strike, BMA Tells Them It's Not Their Fault If People Die. *The Telegraph*, April 26. http://www.telegraph.co.uk/news/2016/04/25/bma-its-not-doctors-fault-if-people-die/.

Dribbusch, Heiner. 2011. Organisieren am Konflikt: Zum Verhältnis von Streik und Mitgliederentwicklung. In *Gewerkschaftliche Modernisierung*, edited by Thomas Haipeter and Klaus Dörre, 231–263. Wiesbaden: VS Verlag.

Esping-Andersen, Gøsta. 1999. *Social Foundations of Postindustrial Economies*. New York: Oxford University Press.

Eurostat. 2016a. Healthcare Provision Statistics. http://ec.europa.eu/eurostat/statistics-explained/index.php/Healthcare_provision_statistics.

Eurostat. 2016b. Healthcare Resource Statistics – Beds. http://ec.europa.eu/eurostat/statistics-explained/index.php/Healthcare_resource_statistics_-_beds#Further_Eurostat_information.

Field, Robert I. 2014. *Mother of Invention: How the Government Created Free-Market Health Care*. Oxford/New York: Oxford University Press.

Foster, Deborah, and Peter Scott. 1998. Conceptualising Union Responses to Contracting Out Municipal Services, 1979–97. *Industrial Relations Journal* no. 29 (2):137–150.

Franke, Detlef Hans. 2007. *Krankenhaus-Management im Umbruch: Konzepte – Methoden - Projekte*. Stuttgart: Kohlhammer.

Galetto, Manuela, Paul Marginson, and Catherine Spieser. 2014. Collective Bargaining and Reforms to Hospital Healthcare Provision: A Comparison of the UK, Italy and France. *European Journal of Industrial Relations* no. 20 (2):131–147.

Geddes, Barbara. 2003. *Paradigms and Sand Castles: Theory Building and Research Design in Comparative Politics*. Ann Arbor: The University of Michigan Press.

Gerlinger, Thomas. 2014. Gesundheitsreform in Deutschland: Hintergrund und jüngere Entwicklungen. In *20 Jahre Wettbewerb im Gesundheitswesen: Theoretische und empirische Analysen zur Ökonomisierung von Medizin und Pflege*, edited by Alexandra Manzei and Rudi Schmiede, 35–44. Wiesbaden: Springer VS.

Gerring, John. 2007. *Case Study Research: Principles and Practices*. Cambridge: Cambridge University Press.

Givan, Rebecca K., and Stephen Bach. 2007. Workforce Responses to the Creeping Privatization of the UK National Health Service. *International Labor and Working-Class History* no. 71 (01):133–153.

Glassner, Vera, Susanne Pernicka, and Nele Dittmar. 2015. *Arbeitsbeziehungen im Krankenhaussektor, Project Report*. Linz: University of Linz.

Gordon, Suzanne. 2009. Institutional Obstacles to Rn Unionization: How 'Vote No' Thinking Is Deeply Embedded in the Nursing Profession. *WorkingUSA* no. 12 (2):279–297.

Greer, Ian. 2008. Social Movement Unionism and Social Partnership in Germany: The Case of Hamburg's Hospitals. *Industrial Relations* no. 47 (4):602–624.

Greer, Ian, and Virginia Doellgast. 2017. Marketization, Inequality, and Institutional Change: Toward a New Framework for Comparative Employment Relations. *Journal of Industrial Relations* no. 59 (2):192–208.

Greer, Ian, Thorsten Schulten, and Nils Böhlke. 2013. How Does Market Making Affect Industrial Relations? Evidence from Eight German Hospitals. *British Journal of Industrial Relations* no. 51 (2):215–239.

Greer, Scott L. 2004. *Territorial Politics and Health Policy: UK Health Policy in Comparative Perspective*. Manchester and New York: Manchester University Press.

Griffiths, Peter, Chiara Dall'Ora, Michael Simon, Jane Ball, Rikard Lindqvist, Anne-Marie Rafferty, Lisette Schoonhoven, Carol Tishelman, and Linda H. Aiken. 2014. Nurses' Shift Length and Overtime Working in 12 European Countries: The Association with Perceived Quality of Care and Patient Safety. *Medical Care* no. 52 (11):975–981.

Griffiths, Roy. 1983. Griffiths Report. http://www.nhshistory.net/griffiths.html.

Grimshaw, Damian. 2009. Can More Inclusive Wage-Setting Institutions Improve Low-Wage Work? Pay Trends in the United Kingdom's Public-Sector Hospitals. *International Labour Review* no. 148 (4):439–459.

Grimshaw, Damian, Karen Jaehrling, Marc van der Meer, Philippe Méhaut, and Nirit Shimron. 2007. Convergent and Divergent Country Trends in Coordinated Wage Setting and Collective Bargaining in the Public Hospitals Sector. *Industrial Relations Journal* no. 38 (6):591–613.

Grimshaw, Damien, Steve Vincent, and Hugh Willmott. 2002. Going Privately: Partnership and Outsourcing in UK Public Services. *Public Administration* no. 80 (3):475–502.

Gruber, Jonathan, and Samuel A. Kleiner. 2012. Do Strikes Kill? Evidence from New York State. *American Economic Journal: Economic Policy* no. 4 (1):127–157.

Halbwachs, Maurice. 1985. *Das Gedächtnis und seine sozialen Bedingungen*. Berlin: suhrkamp.

Hall, Peter A., and David Soskice. 2001. An Introduction to Varieties of Capitalism. In *Varieties of Capitalism. The Institutional Foundations of Comparative Advantage*, edited by Peter A. Hall and David Soskice, 1–71. New York: Oxford University Press.

Heins, Elke, and Richard Parry. 2011. The Role of Wage Bargaining Partners in Public Sector Reform: The Case of Primary Care Contracts. *European Journal of Industrial Relations* no. 17 (4):381–396.

Hellowell, Mark. 2015. Analysis: Borrowing to Save: Can NHS Bodies Ease Financial Pressures by Terminating PFI Contracts? *BMJ*. http //www.bmj.com/bmj/section-pdf/903129/6.

Holst, Hajo. 2013. 'Commodifying Institutions': Vertical Disintegration and Institutional Change in German Labour Relations. *Work, Employment & Society* no. May 23, 2013:1–18.

IAQ. 2019. Beitragssatzentwicklung in der GKV und Anteil der GKV-Ausgaben am BIP 1980–2018. http://www.sozialpolitik-aktuel.de/tl_files/sozialpolitik-aktuell/_Politikfelder/Gesundheitswesen/Datensammlung/PDF-Dateien/abbVI23.pdf.

ISSP Research Group. 2008. International Social Survey Programme: Role of Government IV – ISSP 2006. In *ZA4700 Data file Version 1.0.0*, edited by GESIS Data Archive. Cologne.

Jennings, Karen, and Glenda Western. 1997. A Right to Strike?. *Nursing Ethics* no. 4 (4):277–282.

King's Fund. 2014. Health Select Committee Inquiry into Public Expenditure on Health and Social Care: Evidence from the King's Fund. https://www.kingsfund.org.uk/sites/files/kf/field/field_publication_file/health-select-committee-evidence-public-expenditure-on-health-and-social-care-nov14.pdf.

Klammer, Ute, Christina Klenner, and Sarah Lillemeier. 2018. "Comparable Worth". Arbeitsbewertungen als Blinder Fleck in der Ursachenanalyse des Gender Pay Gaps? Düsseldorf: Hans Böckler Stiftung. https://www.boeckler.de/pdf/p_wsi_studies_14_2018.pdf.

Klein, Rudolf. 2006. *The New Politics of the NHS: From Creation to the Reinvention*. 5th edition. Abingdon: Radcliffe Publishing.

Klenk, Tanja. 2011. Ownership Change and the Rise of a For-Profit Hospital Industry in Germany. *Policy Studies* no. 32 (3):263–275.

Krachler, Nick, and Ian Greer. 2015. When Does Marketisation Lead to Privatisation? Profit-Making in English Health Services after the 2012 Health and Social Care Act. *Social Science & Medicine* no. 124:215–223.

Krämer, Birgit. 2011. Germany: Industrial Relations in the Health Care Sector. http://www.eurofound.europa.eu/eiro/studies/tn1008022s/de1008029q.htm.

Kuehn, Bridget M. 2007. Global Shortage of Health Workers, Brain Drain Stress Developing Countries. *JAMA* no. 298 (16):1853–1855.

Lafer, Gordon. 2005. Hospital Speedups and the Fiction of a Nursing Shortage. *Labor Studies Journal* no. 30 (1):27–46.

Le Grand, Julian. 1991. Quasi-Markets and Social Policy. *The Economic Journal* no. 101:1256–1267.

Lethbridge, Jane. 2011. Public Sector 'Ethos'. In *Working for the State - Employment Relations in the Public Services*, edited by Susan Corby and Graham Symon, 66–83. New York: Palgrave Macmillan.

Lethbridge, Jane. 2012. *Empty Promises: The Impact of Outsourcing on the Delivery of NHS Services, Technical Report*. London: UNISON.

Leys, Colin, and Stewart Player. 2011. *The Plot against the NHS*. Pontypool: Merlin Press.

Lintern, Shaun. 2017a. New Fears Over Nursing Workforce Shortages Revealed. *Healthcare Service Journal*. https://www.hsj.co.uk/topics/workforce/new-fears-over-nursing-workforce-shortages-revealed/7017958.article?blocktitle=Nursing-news&contentID=1745.

Lintern, Shaun. 2017b. Revealed: The Hospitals with the Worst Nurse Staffing. *Nursing Times*. https://www.nursingtimes.net/news/workforce/revealed-the-hospitals-with-the-worst-nurse-staffing/7014987.article.

Littig, Beate. 2011. Expert Interviews. In *International Encyclopedia of Political Science*, edited by Bertrand Badie, Dirk Berg-Schlosser and Leonardo Morlino, 1343–1346. Thousand Oaks: SAGE.

Locke, Richard M., and Kathleen Thelen. 1995. Apples and Oranges Revisited: Contextualized Comparisons and the Study of Comparative Labor Politics. *Politics & Society* no. 23 (2):337–367.

Lutz, Sandy, and E. Preston Gee. 1998. *Columbia/HCA. Healthcare on Overdrive*. New York: McGraw-Hill.

Maarse, Hans. 2006. The Privatisation of Health Care in Europe: An Eight-Country Analysis. *Journal of Health Politics, Policy and Law* no. 31 (5):982–1014.

Marrs, Kira. 2007. Ökonomisierung gelungen, Pflegekräfte wohlauf? *WSI-Mitteilungen* no. 60 (9):502–507.

Mayring, Philipp. 2008. *Qualitative Inhaltsanalyse*. Vol. 10. neu ausgestattete Ausgabe. Weinheim und Basel: Beltz.

Milne, Robin, and Robert Wright. 2004. Competition and Costs: Evidence from Competitive Tendering in the Scottish National Health Service. *Scottish Journal of Political Economy* no. 51 (1):1–23.

Moody, Kim. 2014. Competition and Conflict: Union Growth in the US Hospital Industry. *Economic and Industrial Democracy* no. 35 (1):5–25.

National Audit Office. 2004. *Improving Patient Care by Reducing the Risk of Hospital Acquired Infection: A Progress Report*. London: The Stationery Office.

National Audit Office. 2011. Achievement of Foundation Trust Status by NHS Hospital Trusts. London: National Audit Office. https://www.nao.org.uk/wp-content/uploads/2011/10/10121516.pdf.

National Audit Office. 2014a. The Financial Sustainability of NHS Bodies. London: National Audit Office.

National Audit Office. 2014b. Monitor: Regulating NHS foundation trusts. London: National Audit Office.

Naylor, Chris, and Sarah Gregory. 2009. Briefing: Independent Sector Treatment Centres. http://www.kingsfund.org.uk/sites/files/kf/field/field_publication_file/briefing-independent-sector-treatment-centres-istc-chris-naylor-sarah-gregory-kings-fund-october-2009.pdf.

NHS. 2017. About the National Health Service. https://www.nhs.uk/NHSEngland/thenhs/about/Pages/overview.aspx.

Obinger, Herbert, Carina Schmitt, and Stefan Traub. 2016. *The Political Economy of Privatization in Rich Democracies*. Oxford: Oxford University Press.

OECD. 2017. Statistics Database. Health, Health Care Resources, Hospitals. https://stats.oecd.org/Index.aspx?DataSetCode=HEALTH_REAC.

OECD. 2019. *Health at a Glance 2019: OECD Indicators*. Paris: OECD Publishing. https://doi.org/10.1787/4dd50c09-en.

OECD. 2020a. Health Care Resources. https://stats.oecd.org/index.aspx?queryid=30183#.

OECD. 2020b. Health Care Utilisation. https://stats.oecd.org/Index.aspx?DataSetCode=HEALTH_PROC.

OECD. 2020c. Health Expenditure and Financing. https://stats.oecd.org/Index.aspx?DataSetCode=SHA

Pillinger, Jane. 2010. Pay and the Gender Wage Gap in Health and Social Care. Report of EPSU Study on Pay in the Care Sector in Relation to Overall Pay Levels and the Gender Pay Gap in Different Countries in the European Union. *EPSU*. http://www.epsu.org/article/report-pay-and-gender-wage-gap-health-and-social-care.

Pollock, Allyson. 2003. Foundation Hospitals Will Kill the NHS. *The Guardian*, May 7. https://www.theguardian.com/politics/2003/may/07/publicservices.comment.

Pollock, Allyson. 2004. *NHS plc: The Privatisation of Our Healthcare*. London: Verso.

Pollock, Allyson M., David Price, Alison Talbot-Smith, and John Mohan. 2003. NHS and the Health and Social Care Bill: End of Bevan's Vision?. *BMJ* no. 327 (7421):982–985.

Pond, Richard. 2006. Liberalisation, Privatisation and Regulation in the UK Healthcare Sector/Hospitals. http://www.pique.at/reports/pubs/PIQUE_CountryReports_Health_UK_November2006.pdf.

Propper, Carol, and Will Bartlett. 1997. The Impact of Competition on the Behaviour of National Health Service Trusts. In *Contracting for Health: Quasi-Markets and the National Health Service*, edited by Robert Flynn and Gareth Williams, 14–29. Oxford: Oxford University Press.

Prosser, Thomas. 2011. UK: Industrial Relations in the Health Care Sector. http://www.eurofound.europa.eu/eiro/studies/tn1008022s/uk1008029q.html.

Przeworski, Adam, and Henry Teune. 1970. *The Logic of Comparative Social Inquiry*. New York: Wiley-Interscience.

Quaglio, GianLuca, Theodoros Karapiperis, Lieve Van Woensel, Elleke Arnold, and David McDaid. 2013. Austerity and Health in Europe. *Health Policy* no. 113 (1):13–19. https://doi.org/10.1016/j.healthpol.2013.09.005.

RCN. 2014. An Uncertain Future: The UK Nursing Labour Market Review 2014. https:// www2.rcn.org.uk/__data/assets/pdf_file/0005/597713/004_740.pdf.

RCN. 2020. Pat Cullen Nominated for Prestigious Award for Leading Nurses in Unprecedented Strike Action. https://www.rcn.org.uk/news-and-events/news/pat-cullen-nominated-for-prestigious-award-for-leading-nurses-in-unprecedented-strike-action.

Reich, Adam. 2012. *With God on Our Side. The Struggle for Workers' Rights in a Catholic Hospital*. Ithaca/London: ILR Press.

Roderick, Peter, and Allyson Pollock. 2014. A Wolf in Sheep's Clothing: How Monitor is Using Licensing Powers to Reduce Hospital and Community Services in England under the Guise of Continuity. BMJ, *349:g5603* http://dx.doi.org/10.1136/bmj.g5603.

Rohlfing, Ingo. 2012. *Case Studies and Causal Inference: An Integrative Framework*. Basingstoke: Palgrave Macmillan. https://books.google.de/books?id=7T7R2BCebtEC.

Rothgang, Heinz, Mirella Cacace, Simone Grimmeisen, and Claus Wendt. 2005. The Changing Role of the State in Healthcare Systems. *European Review* no. 13 (Supplement S1):187–212.

Schreyögg, Jonas. 2016. Expertise zur Ermittlung des Zusammenhangs zwischen Pflegeverhältniszahlen und pflegesensitiven Ergebnisparametern in Deutschland im Auftrag des Bundesministeriums für Gesundheit (BMG). https://www.bundesgesundheitsministerium.de/fileadmin/Dateien/5_Publikationen/Pflege/Berichte/Gutachten_Schreyoegg_Pflegesensitive_Fachabteilungen.pdf.

Schulten, Thorsten. 2006. Liberalisation, Privatisation and Regulation in the German Healthcare Sector/Hospitals. *PIQUE Research Report*. http://www.boeckler.de/pdf/wsi_pj_piq_sekkrankh.pdf.

Schulten, Thorsten, and Nils Böhlke. 2009. Die Privatisierung von Krankenhäusern in Deutschland und ihre Auswirkung auf Beschäftigte und Patienten. In *Privatisierung von Krankenhäusern. Gegenstrategien aus gewerkschaftlicher und zivilgesellschaftlicher Perspektive*, edited by Nils Böhlke, Thomas Gerlinger, Kai Mosebach, Rolf Schmucker and Thorsten Schulten, 97–123. Hamburg: VSA.

Schwartz, Hermann. 2001. Round Up the Usual Suspects!: Globalization, Domestic Politics, and Welfare State Change. In *The New Politics of the Welfare State*, edited by Paul Pierson, 17–44. Oxford: Oxford University Press.

Schwierz, Christoph. 2011. Expansion in Markets with Decreasing Demand-For-Profits in the German Hospital Industry. *Health Economics* no. 20:675–687.

Schweizer, Lars, and Barbara Bernhard. 2009. Strategische Optionen öffentlicher Krankenhäuser zwischen Markt und Hierarchie – Eine empirische Studie. In *Vernetzung im Gesundheitswesen: Wettbewerb und Kooperation*, edited by Volker E. Amelung, Jörg Sydow and Arnold Windeler. Stuttgart: Kohlhammer.

Scott, W. Richard, Martin Ruef, Peter J. Mendel, and Carol A. Caronna. 2000. *Institutional Change and Healthcare Organizations: From Professional Dominance to Managed Care*. Chicago/London: The University of Chicago Press.

Scourfield, Peter. 2016. Squaring the Circle: What Lessons Can Be Learned from the Hinchingbrooke Franchise Fiasco?. *Critical Social Policy* no. 36 (1):142–152.

Simon, Michael. 2007a. Das Deutsche DRG-Fallpauschalensystem: Kritische Anmerkungen zu Begründungen und Zielen. *Jahrbuch für kritische Medizin* no. 44:41–63.

Simon, Michael. 2007b. Stellenabbau im Pflegedienst der Krankenhäuser: Eine Analyse der Entwicklung zwischen 1991 und 2005. *efh-papers* (P07-001). http://serwiss.bib.hs-hannover.de/frontdoor/index/index/docId/60.

Simon, Michael. 2020. Das DRG-Fallpauschalensystem für Krankenhäuser. Kritische Bestandsaufnahme und Eckpunkte für eine Reform der Krankenhausfinanzierung jenseits des DRG-Systems. *Working Paper Forschungsförderung der Hans-Böckler-Stiftung* no. No. 196, November.

Stabile, Mark, Sarah Thomson, Sara Allin, SSéan Boyle, Reinhard Busse, Karine Chevreul, Greg Marchildon, and Elias Mossialos. 2013. Health Care Cost Containment Strategies Used in Four Other High-Income Countries Hold Lessons for the United States. *Health Affairs* no. 32 (4):643–652.

Statistisches Bundesamt. 2015. *Gesundheit: Kostennachweis der Krankenhäuser, Fachserie 12 Reihe 6.3 - 2015*. Wiesbaden: Statistisches Bundesamt.

Statistisches Bundesamt. 2017. Gesundheit – Ausgaben. In *Fachserie 12, Reihe 7.1.1*. Statistisches Bundesamt. https://www.destatis.de/DE/Publikationen/Thematisch/ Gesundheit/Gesundheitsausgaben/AusgabenGesundheitPDF_2120711.pdf; jsessionid=F25386D238A268639BACE52B290123ED.cae2?__blob=publicationFile.

Statistisches Bundesamt. 2020a. Gesundheitsausgabenrechnung. http://www.gbe-bund.de/.

Statistisches Bundesamt. 2020b. Krankenhausstatistik – Grunddaten der Krankenhäuser und Vorsorge- oder Rehabilitationseinrichtungen. https://www.gbe-bund.de/gbe/ abrechnung.prc_abr_test_logon?p_uid=gast&p_aid=0&p_knoten=FID&p_ sprache=D&p_suchstring=411.

Tailby, Stephanie. 2012. Public Service Restructuring in the UK: The Case of the English National Health Service. *Industrial Relations Journal* no. 43 (5):448–464.

U.S. Department of Health and Human Services. 2008. Discharges and Days of Care from the National Hospital Discharge Survey. http://www.cdc.gov/nchs/nhds/ nhds_publications.htm#nhds.

U.S. Department of Health and Human Services. 2010. The Registered Nurse Population: Findings from the 2008 National Sample Survey of Registered Nurses. http://bhpr.hrsa. gov/healthworkforce/rnsurveys/rnsurveyfinal.pdf.

UNISON. 2014. UNISON TUPE Branch Guidance. https://www.unison.org.uk/content/ uploads/2014/04/On-line-Catalogue223172.pdf.

UNISON. 2016. UNISON Annual Report 2015/16. UNISON. https://www.unison.org. uk/content/uploads/2016/04/23784.pdf.

UNISON. 2017a. About. https://www.unison.org.uk/about/.

UNISON. 2017b. How Much Does It Cost to Be a UNISON Member? https://join. unison.org.uk/membership-rates/.

UNISON. 2017c. UNISON: Stronger Together. Annual Report 2016/17. UNISON. https://www.unison.org.uk/content/uploads/2017/C5/UNISONAnnual-Report-2017. pdf.

ver.di. 2003. *Aus:Wertung Gesundheitskampgne – Erkentnisse und Erfahrungen zur Kampagnenarbeit in ver.di*. Berlin: ver.di.

ver.di. 2015a. Bundesweiter Nachtdienstcheck: Deutsche Krankenhäuser zum Teil gefährlich unterbesetzt. https://www.verdi.de/themen/nachrichten/++co++4ee62322-c3e5-11e4-9073-5254008a33df.

ver.di. 2015b. Mehr von uns ist besser für alle: Geschäftsbericht Fachbereich 3, 1. Januar 2011 bis 31. Dezember 2014. Berlin. https://gesundheit-soziales.verdi. de/++file++5530938e6f68447bc90010a5/download/Gesch%C3%A4ftsbericht_ Fachbereich%203_20150309.pdf.

ver.di. 2019a. Entlastung per Tarifvertrag. https://gesundheit-soziales.verdi.de/ ++file++5d8df7de2d9efb1409d75633/download/Brosch%C3%BCre%20Tarifvertrag-Entlastung-2019.pdf.

ver.di. 2019b. Geschäftsbericht Bundesfachbereich Gesundheit, Soziale Dienste, Wohlfahrt und Kirchen. https://gesundheit-soziales.verdi.de/++file++5e287177bc91d0b31f5447c6/download/2018_Gesch%C3%A4ftsbericht-FB3_SCREEN.pdf.

ver.di. 2020. DKG, DPR und ver.di verständigen sich auf Pflegepersonalbedarfsbemessung sinstrument – Neue Vorgaben sollen bedarfsgerechte Pflege sichern. https://www.verdi.de/presse/pressemitteilungen/++co++83affd32-36b1-11ea-a602-525400b665de.

Walness, Derek. 2002. *Securing Our Future Health: Taking a Long-Term View*. London: HM Treasury.

Watt, Nicholas. 2014. Income from Private Patients Soars at NHS Hospital Trusts *The Guardian*, August 19. https://www.theguardian.com/society/2014/aug/19/private-patient-income-soars-nhs-privatisation.

Wehkamp, Karl-Heinz, and Heinz Naegler. 2017. The Commercialization of Patient-Related Decision Making in Hospitals: A Qualitative Study of the Perceptions of Doctors and Chief Executive Officers. *Deutsches Ärzteblatt International* no. 114 (47):797.

White, Joseph. 2007. Markets and Medical Care: The United States, 1993-2005. *The Milbank Quarterly* no. 85 (3):395–448.

Whitfield, Dexter. 2006. A Typology of Privatisation and Marketisation. *ESSU Research Report No. 1*. https://www.european-services-strategy.org.uk/wp-content/uploads/2006/11/essu-research-paper-1-2.pdf.

Wolf, Luigi. 2015. Mehr von uns ist besser für alle: die Streiks an der Berliner Charité und ihre Bedeutung für die Aufwertung von Care-Arbeit. In *UMCARE: Gesundheit und Pflege neu organisieren*, edited by Barbara Fried and Hannah Schurian, 23–31. Berlin: Rosa-Luxemburg-Stiftung.

2 Marketization, opportunity structures, and local-level determinants of trade union action

2.1 Introduction

The question to be answered in this chapter is, how can the choice of trade union strategies in times of marketization be analyzed, and what are its main determinants? Traditional comparative industrial relations research usually starts from the Varieties of Capitalism (VoC) typology that characterizes differences in the production systems of liberal and coordinated market economies. VoCs, however, were not designed with regard to public services and fail to acknowledge institutional dynamics, especially in times of liberalization, as well as local-level variation. This book therefore draws on approaches that take institutional dynamics into account and complements them with concepts relevant to local-level variation.

2.2 Macro-institutional theories

2.2.1 Varieties of capitalism

In order to explain differences in trade union behavior, traditional industrial relations literature usually draws on the VoC approach (Hall and Soskice 2001). The approach distinguishes between the coordinated market economy (CME) type and the liberal market economy type (LME). According to this typology, the German market economy is characterized by high value-added and skill-dependent manufacturing industries that for their success rely on company- or industry-specific skills, innovation, and collaboration between firms. The labor market is less mobile and employment less subject to competition. Labor relations in this system are cooperative and characterized by institutionalized inclusion of employees through codetermination, collective bargaining, and social dialogue. Trade union density is typically high, and employers cooperate and organize themselves into associations. This way, collective bargaining is relatively centralized. By contrast, Great Britain is a LME based on competitive markets and at-will employment. The labor market is dependent on general skills and flexible, short-term, and deregulated employment. Low trade union density and limited coordination of employers in associations characterizes labor relations in this system. Accordingly, collective bargaining is relatively decentralized (Hall and Soskice 2001).

The two ideal types are reinforced by under what is known as institutional complementarities. Historically, it was not due to labor strength that CME institutions emerged, but due to cross-class coalitions and employer support. Institutions are complementary in the sense that, in both systems, employers have a stake in maintaining the national labor relations institutions, because employers organized their production around these institutions to gain competitive advantages. This causes diverging trends that stabilize the institutional systems. Due to these historical roots, these systems have not fundamentally changed in times of globalization and crisis. Moreover, the relevant level of analysis here consists of national institutions that create incentives which structure the subnational and local practices of actors. In this sense, the national level determines practices on lower levels (Mares 2000; Palier and Thelen 2010).

Accordingly, a VoC approach postulates that common market pressures would not have a transformative effect, unless they change national labor relations institutions. Observable changes are mere modifications that do not only undermine coordination but even stabilize it under the new prevailing conditions (Hall and Soskice 2001; Hall and Gingerich 2009). Thus, political economy processes, such as marketization, might modify coordination but still reinforce the distinctiveness of LMEs and CMEs. Furthermore, VoC postulates differing responses by unions to competitive pressures. In Germany, "adequate institutional supports" (Baccaro, Hamann, and Turner 2003, 119) create a disincentive to "mobilize their membership [...] build coalitions with other groups, or give support to grass-roots initiatives" (p. 121), whereas British unions compensate for a weak institutional position by building coalitions and mobilizing members (ibid.).

2.2.2 *Liberalization theory*

Researchers analyzing liberalization trends contest the view of the reproduction of institutions that implies only gradual change. They underline that capitalism is inherently dynamic and not well captured by notions of stable equilibria, path dependence, coordination problems, and neat institutional regulation. Studying national labor relations institutions alongside broader political economy processes, they perceive liberalizing trends as an erosion of the arrangements that have characterized CMEs. These scholars claim that market economies are now tending toward more commonalities than differences because market economies are adaptive and liberalization is deeply transformative, so the CMEs today are converging upon the logic of LMEs (Glyn 2006; Howell 2006; Streeck 2009; Baccaro and Howell 2011). This way, Katz and Darbishire (2000) focus on the common trend of liberalization of employment patterns in the telecommunications and automotive industries since the 1980s. They find variation within countries, but much commonality across most different countries is in the nature of that variation and the processes through which variation is appearing. Also, Bordogna (2008) found that structural pressures to compete, liberalize, and undermine worker power serve to diminish the protective effects that national labor relations institutions may afford. This is also the case for public sector employment relations because new public management reforms necessitate a transformation of employment relations toward less job security.

Baccaro and Howell (2011) argue that this change in employment relations does not necessarily depend on a change in formal institutions. They showed that employment relations regimes in rich democracies have not changed in terms of their institutional forms but have modified their *functions* in a convergent direction, namely toward greater employer discretion through institutional deregulation. This is what they call plasticity of political-economic institutions: the capacity of institutions to function quite differently in new contexts. The authors conclude that the focus on institutional forms is likely to overlook the malleability of institutions. Institutions can appear unchanged but in fact perform in different ways than before. However, continued differences in institutional forms can be perfectly compatible with convergence in institutional function. Institutions will then perform in a similar fashion and generate similar outcomes, which will lead to a convergent trajectory of institutional performance across different countries. Despite different starting points and paces of change, they find clear evidence for a common neoliberal directionality to institutional change in employment relations. The authors conclude that this also raises questions about the centrality of institutions in comparative political economy research. Instead, they suggest directing more attention to the plasticity of institutional functioning and the transformative power of incremental change (Baccaro and Howell 2011).

Given the profound marketization processes outlined in Chapter 1, which are comparable to each other and even more pronounced in Germany than in England, as well as the employment relations characteristics, the VoC approach does not seem to appropriately capture the dynamics and specificities of the health sector. The framework does not generally match the experience of public sector unions (Bach and Bordogna 2011). The original focus of the VoC framework was on social security systems and their consequences for wage earners, and it has proved difficult to apply the framework to health systems, in part because of the strong role of public sector health services in Britain's allegedly liberal regime (Bambra 2005). Also, the characterization of British and German unions' responses to competitive pressures of liberalization theory is inconsistent with what has been observed in the studies presented. Therefore, in the following section, analytical approaches that consider institutional dynamics and (local level) agency will be highlighted.

2.3 Process-oriented approach

2.3.1 Institutional dynamics and trade unionism

As discussed in the previous section, welfare state and employment relations institutions are inherently dynamic. Greer and Doellgast (2017) describe two mechanisms through which marketization drives institutional change that is marked by an increase in economic and social inequality. The first mechanism is the shift of managers and investors from voice to exit: Instead of seeking influence via negotiation and compromise, managers and investors threaten to avoid the institutions of employment relations or labor market protection by shifting production or services to other countries. Public employers can exit by means of privatization and outsourcing. Thus, they undermine traditional participative structures and the corresponding labor power, which leads to a disorganization of industrial relations and welfare provision institutions (Greer and Doellgast 2017, 198 f.). The second mechanism is a shift from productive toward nonproductive economic activities, since intensified competition increases market uncertainty and constrains profit margins of productive economic activities. This leads to an increase of professional services that derive profits mainly from exchange-based activities, such as those found in models of public–private partnerships or privatization in the public sector. This shift increases pressure to change the corresponding regulations in the financial, labor, and public tendering domains to further support profit extraction that creates new forms of undemocratic private and public regulation of markets, insulated from public scrutiny (Greer and Doellgast 2017, 200 f.).

The two mechanisms lead to economic inequality since they increase the share of income going to capital and the share of government transfers going to financial institutions. Moreover, they foster growth of low-wage and insecure jobs, leading to earnings dispersion. Both exit strategies also have transformative effects for employment relations. They are accompanied by leaving the employers' association, remaining nonunion, adopting precarious contracts, using collective agreements from other sectors with lower standards, etc. Social inequality increases through declining collective power and voice of workers, as well as shrinking transparency and scope for democratic public debate on these policies (Greer and Doellgast 2017, 202 f.).

A model that takes into account dynamics of institutional change is Frege and Kelly's (2003) Social Movement Model of Union Strategic Choice (see Figure 2.1). In this model, trade unions are actors that can choose from a set of strategies. This choice is influenced by various interdependent factors. It starts from social and economic changes, i.e. changes in economic structures and of labor and product markets. It also considers the institutional context of industrial relations, which includes collective bargaining structures, legal and arbitration procedures as well as the political system. Also, employers and government are treated as actors that pursue different strategies over time and across different countries, influencing unions' strategic choices. Such choices are further influenced by the unions' structure, whether they are organized horizontally or hierarchically, centralized or decentralized, or if the trade union movement is unified or fragmented. These factors are moderated through the process variable of framing, which Frege and Kelly (2003, 14) define as "ways in which unionists perceive and think about changes in their external context as threats or opportunities". The specific framing often depends on the union's identity and their idea of union action, the so-called repertoire of contention.

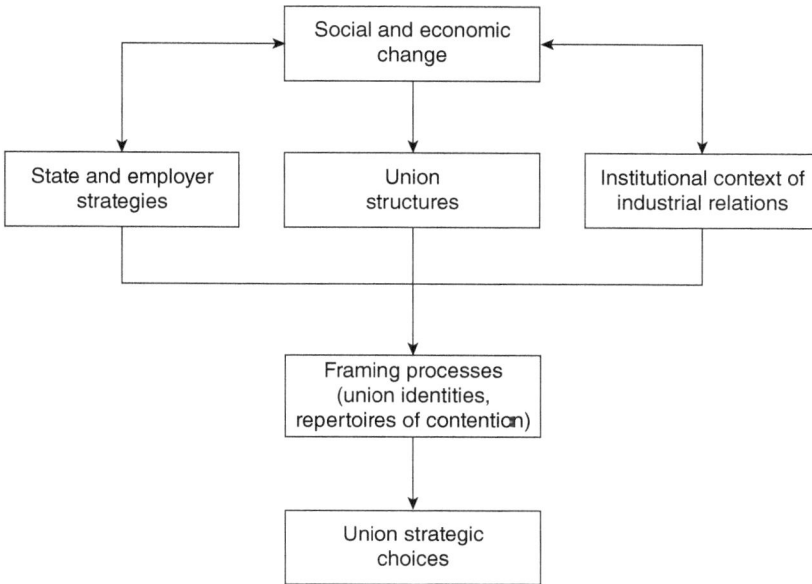

Figure 2.1 A social movement model of union strategic choice.

The theoretical approach of this study will start from this model and the idea of institutional dynamics. Further, it will make additions and specifications to the relevant factors in the Frege and Kelly Model. I will expand, in particular, on opportunity structures, as well as local-level and agency factors that determine trade union strategies and their leeway for action.

2.3.2 Political opportunities brought about by institutional dynamics

As discussed above and in contrast to the path dependency emphasized by VoC, political economy processes can lead to radical changes over short periods (Hauptmeier 2012, 740). Political economy processes have effects on and interact with national labor relations institutions. This can of course put unions in a defensive position, leading them to make concessions, and ultimately facing the exit of disappointed members (Hirschman 1970). At the same time, opportunity structures may allow actors to make use of social change processes, leading to a radical change. Frege and Kelly (2003) include the perception of external context changes as threats or opportunities as a process variable that influences trade union strategic choices. Other authors elaborated further on the emergence and potential of political opportunities, and will be presented below to further examine this factor.

Crucial for a political opportunity to arise and be exploited is the salience of the issue of interest. A highly politically salient issue is defined as one of "importance to the average voter, relative to other political issues" (Culpepper 2010, 4). Culpepper explains how legislation and regulation affecting the business environment, especially if they evolve around highly technical economic issues, often serve the interest of corporations and business organizations. These issues are of low political salience and political parties will only increase their expertise in these fields if the topic is highly visible and of interest to their voters. Issues of abstract and technical character and without direct effect on voters are especially difficult for voters to comprehend and political parties have no incentive to increase voters' knowledge in order to win elections. In this low salience environment, business will succeed due to superior lobbying capacities and "deference of legislators and reporters toward managerial expertise" (Culpepper 2010, 4 ff.). This effect is reinforced by the media that tends to report on topics of high salience. Regarding low salience topics, business can use its "informational asymmetries" vis-à-vis politicians, and its acknowledged expertise to frame press coverage. This is what Culpepper calls "quiet politics" (Culpepper 2010, 10).

However, business influence is fragile since it is only "a function of public inattention" (Culpepper 2010, 178) and their weapons lose effect if the topic comes to public attention. When salience increases and an issue becomes of public interest, voters gain interest in and knowledge about it, politicians start caring about public opinion and disregard powerful business groups. When salience is low, the public does not matter rather the perception of superior expertise on the part of business groups and their access to decision-makers. When salience increases, business has to persuade the public as well. This means that "the more the public cares about an issue, the less managerial organizations will be able to exercise disproportionate influence over the rules governing that issue", or, in short, "business power goes down as political salience goes up" (Culpepper 2010, 177). Political salience can increase under two circumstances: market crashes that reveal failure of managers or business expertise, and scandals. Both can be used to mobilize the public, especially when the issue is associated with widely shared values such as clean air, pure water, or health and safety. Media will again reinforce this effect by increasingly reporting on the issue, creating incentives for politicians to acquire expertise, and adjusting their positions regarding the highly salient issue (Culpepper 2010, 6 ff.).

Increasingly salient topics can change power structures and create political opportunities. Ganz (2000, 1019) calls these political opportunities "focal moments", which reconfigure leadership and organizations, and can create dramatically new strategic possibilities, including conditions. "Opportunities often occur at moments of unusual structural fluidity" (Ganz 2009, 9), i.e., at moments combining uncertainty with significance. In these moments, opportunities do not arise because actors acquire more resources, but because existing resources acquire more value (Ganz 2009).

One example of radical political economy changes that create opportunity structures is the disintegration of the German labor relations system through workforce dualization (Hassel 1999), as well as vertical disintegration (Doellgast and Greer 2007). Because of legislative changes in the early 2000s that permitted a greater use of temporary agency work, and the fact that codetermination does not allow workers any say with regard to the use of temporary agency work or outsourcing of production, German managers in the automotive and telecommunications industries have made extensive use of these tools to deal with increased international competition (Doellgast and Greer 2007, 71). In addition, the metalworkers' union also chose to focus on job security over workers' rights during the great financial crisis, leading to a dualization of the workforce into core permanent and peripheral temporary workers (Hassel 2014). In this way, within a decade, the German labor relations system has faced significant changes resembling more liberal forms of labor relations, including the healthcare sector (Greer, Schulten, and Böhlke 2013).

Furthermore, again in contrast to the VoC approach that assumes that national institutions have direct effects on actors' practices, other authors argue that "there is a gap between institutional rules and their enactment" (Streeck and Thelen 2005) from which political opportunities can arise as well. This gap gives actors "some leeway in deciding" (Behrens, Hamann, and Hurd 2004, 24) how they want to focus their resources and make use of opportunities to actively shape outcomes. One example is the renegotiation of national and workplace employment relations institutions in the German construction sector due to transnational subcontracting (Wagner 2015). Another example is the differences in how the same national employment relations institutions in Spain played out on the firm level due to differences in actors' ideologies (Hauptmeier 2012).

Crucial to the use of these opportunity structures is, according to Nachtwey and Wolf (2013, 106 f.), the capability to act ("Handlungsvermögen"). Unions need to first possess the capability to recognize political opportunity structures on the firm, societal, and political level if they want to use them effectively. Gamson and Meyer (1996) pursued this idea further and argued that political opportunities do not only need to be recognized but agency also needs to be perceived to be potentially successful. An optimistic rhetoric of change and the belief that action can then even create political opportunities, can become a self-fulfilling prophecy (Gamson and Meyer 1996 but also Diani 1996; Goodwin and Jasper 1999).

2.4 Local-level and organizational factors of trade unionism

2.4.1 Local-level variation

The VoC approach, as well as liberalization theory, implicitly assumes a determination of trade union strategies via national system-level factors and generally disregard the local level. Also, Frege and Kelly (2003) focus mainly on national institutional factors that determine unions' strategic choices. However, their model allows for some agency of unions since it accounts for framing processes. This study will place a special focus on agency and local-level determinants of trade union strategies, to extend and elaborate on their model.

As demonstrated by Locke (1992) in his classic study on how union strategy and structure created within-country variation in the Italian automotive sector, trade union strategies and outcomes are not fully determined by national-level factors, but can vary locally. The theoretical approach of this study will use the concepts of power resources and capabilities to explain local-level variation, understood as the use of political opportunities and local trade unions' strategic choices.

Based on what has been theorized above, an extension to the model of strategic union choice of Frege and Kelly (2003) will be suggested. This approach not only builds on the authors' idea that social and economic changes impact unions' strategies but also places a stronger focus on the opportunity structures that marketization processes produce, as well as the resources and capabilities unions possess and can build up to use these political opportunities.

2.4.2 Power resources

When including the recognition of political opportunities and local-level leeway into the model of strategic union choice by Frege and Kelly (2003), unions also need the resources and capabilities to use their agency. Frege and Kelly's (2003) model addresses institutional and structural power resources as part of the institutional context of industrial relations. However, as part of the institutional context, these power resources appear to be broadly structurally determined and can only be influenced by unions to a limited degree. This view has been contested recently, and it is worth taking a closer look at the further developments in power resource theory.

As mentioned above, to use opportunity structures brought about by marketization processes and local-level leeway, unions need to utilize their power emanating from different resources. Lévesque and Murray (2010, 335) describe these resources as "fixed or path-dependent assets that an actor can normally access and mobilize". However, Benassi, Doellgast, and Sarmiento-Mirwaldt (2016) have shown that power resources for labor and capital can change in short periods of time. In this study, I will take this dynamic approach to power resources since unions are acting in a changing environment. Power resources can also be activated, built, and developed in short periods of time if unions possess the appropriate capabilities (also see Section 2.4.3). Traditional power resources theory distinguishes two types of power sources: structural power and associational power.

The concept of associational power refers to the forms of power that result from the organization as a collective actor (Wright 2000; Silver 2003). This is mainly, but not exclusively, reflected in trade union density. The willingness of members to participate actively in the union and in collective action is another important factor for associational power (among others Offe and Wiesenthal 1980). Unions also need sufficient material and personnel resources (Lévesque and Murray 2010, 336 f.) as well as an efficient internal structure to organize and participate in conflicts (Behrens, Hurd, and Waddington 2004). In addition, they need flexibility in the structural organization of the union and reconciliation of members' interests (Ganz 2000), as well as solidarity between members (internal cohesion) (Lévesque and Murray 2010, 336 f.).

Structural power refers to the power resulting from the location of workers within the economic system. It can be further differentiated into the workers' position in the labor market, the so-called marketplace bargaining power, or, in other words, the power that "results directly from tight labor markets". Further, stemming from the workers' position in the process of production, it distinguishes the so-called workplace bargaining power, meaning the power that results "from the strategic location of a particular group of workers within a key industrial sector" (Wright 2000, 962; Silver 2003, 13).

To account specifically for the context of coordinated market economies in continental Europe, these two concepts were complemented by the concept of institutional power. It refers to the power that results from conflicts and negotiations that are based on structural and associational power. It is thus a solidified form of the relative strength of unions and employers. However, it not only grants rights to unions but also restricts their action. The particularity of institutional power is its temporal persistence: it can survive economic changes and short-term changes in societal balances of power, particularly if it is legally regulated. Nevertheless, it can change over time if the economic context changes, if employers change their attitude, or due to legal–political attacks on trade unions' institutional power (Brinkmann et al. 2008, 25; Brinkmann and Nachtwey 2010, 21; Schmalz and Dörre 2014, 230).

Additionally, to account for processes outside of the workplace, the concept of societal power was introduced. It refers to the ability of trade unions to cooperate with and mobilize other civil society actors, as well as to intervene in public discussions and increase pressure or frame societal problems (Ganz 2000, 147 f.; Lévesque and Murray 2013; Schmalz and Dörre 2014, 232). It can be further divided into network power or network embeddedness (Frege, Heery, and Turner 2004; Turner 2006; Lévesque and Murray 2010) and discourse power or narrative resources (Chun 2009; Lévesque and Murray 2010). To separate the network resources from networking capabilities, network embeddedness is defined as the existence of adequate actors in the community for potential networks (Gindin 2016), as well as the density and diversity of existing networks between unions and the community (Lévesque and Murray 2010, 339). In the same way, discourse power is defined only as the potential for public support of a cause, for instance as a strong preference of the public for public healthcare provision. Activating this resource by deploying suitable frames will be treated as a capability.

Regarding the English–German comparison, it is important to point out that in the past the influence of German trade unions was based more on state recognition than on their own associational power. Their associational power was replaced by political institutionalization. Lately, trade unions increasingly use US American strategies of mobilization and organization, such as community organizing or campaigning. This can be explained by a partial loss of their state recognition. Using the US American models in a CME context also means leaving the seemingly institutionally determined path (Brinkmann et al. 2008; Rehder 2014, 252 f.).

The different power resources can also interact with one another. Trade unions have to balance what Schmitter and Streeck (1999) called the "logic of influence", which would be based mostly on institutional power or aim at sustaining or expanding their influence in decision-making processes, and the "logic of membership", which would be based mostly on associational power and aim at increasing trade union density, as well as and enforcing members' interests. The relationship between the different forms of power can in some cases be regarded as a trade-off. For example, unions that have strong institutional power in the form of access to decision-makers, which helps them influence new public management restructuring processes in the hospital sector, are less likely to use their societal power and organize public mobilization (Galetto, Marginson, and Spieser 2014). Conversely, as Greer (2008) has shown in the case of the privatization of hospitals in Hamburg, the erosion of their channels of influence may lead them to develop public campaigning tactics to compensate.

Last, but not least, unions need to be able to understand their own sources of power and use them effectively. Such capability is often lacking (McAlevey 2016). The capabilities necessary to recognize, build, sustain, and deploy resources will be fleshed out in the next section.

2.4.3 Capabilities

This section will present two approaches that distinguish resources and capabilities and will synthesize them to develop a classification of capabilities suitable for extending Frege and Kelly's (2003) model. This extension includes some of the capabilities as understood by the authors that will be reviewed below. Frege and Kelly (2003) mention union structures that refer, among others, to the internal organization of the union, as well as their identity and framing of social and economic change. To extend and specify Frege and Kelly's model, Ganz (2000) on resources and resourcefulness, as well as Lévesque and Murray (2010) on union resources and capabilities will be reviewed. The most relevant capabilities for this study will subsequently be presented in more detail.

From his study of two rival trade unions that were trying to unionize California's farmworkers in the 1960s, Ganz (2000) developed the concept of resources and resourcefulness. In his study, Ganz found that it was not the well-established and The American Federation of Labor and Congress of Industrial Organizations (AFL–CIO)-affiliated Agricultural Workers Organizing Committee, but the newly formed, precariously funded, and independent United Farm Workers that succeeded in organizing Californian farm workers. In contrast to earlier studies that explained different outcomes with a more favorable political opportunity structure or charismatic leadership, Ganz argues that it can be explained by differences in their strategies due to the unions' respective strategic capacity, i.e., their resourcefulness. In times of changing environments, resourcefulness is of particular importance for innovative processes and adjustment to new conditions. The changing conditions can generate opportunities for action, but the outcome depends on how unions use them (Ganz 2009).

According to Ganz (2000), strategic capacity of the leadership of an organization and an organization itself depends on three elements. (1) Salient knowledge refers to relevant information about a domain in which an organization acts. Given changing environments, (2) heuristic processes are important in order to use salient knowledge to adapt to new problems and devise novel solutions. Diversity in the leadership and organization facilitates innovation. Another critical element for creative output is (3) motivation. It will influence actors' focus on their work, their persistence, and ability to sustain high energy, as well as the acquisition of domain-specific knowledge and skills. If actors are intrinsically motivated and thus intensely interested in a problem or dissatisfied with the status quo, their intense occupation with the domain can make them think more critically and reflectively (Ganz 2000, 1011–1014). Trade unions that possess strategic capacities will be more likely to devise effective and creative strategies, with which they can even compensate for a lack of material resources (Ganz 2000, 1041).

Additionally, Lévesque and Murray (2010) stress the importance of strategic capacity – capabilities[1] as they call it – to effectively use power resources in their union power framework. They distinguish between power resources that are, in their view, fixed or path-dependent assets, which actors can access and mobilize, and the more dynamic capabilities that are "sets of aptitudes, competencies, abilities, social skills or know-how that can be developed, transmitted and learned" (Lévesque and Murray 2010, 341). Similar to Ganz, Lévesque and Murray argue that power resources are necessary but not sufficient for successful trade union action since conditions under which unions act are rapidly changing. Accordingly, weakening union power is traced back to a lack in the capability to adapt strategies to changed circumstances. Thus, capabilities are central to developing power resources and successful organizational routines in a changing environment. Lévesque and Murray identify four strategic capabilities. (1) Intermediation refers to the capability of unions to mediate between contending interests, to foster collaborative action, and to access, create, and activate social networks. The capability of (2) framing is characterized by a union's ability to define a proactive and autonomous agenda. It is crucial for extending repertoires of contention and justifying the use of new practices, as well as for mobilization of members and allies. (3) Articulation refers to the global context in which unions operate and their ability to transpose local issues into a larger context and vice versa. Finally, (4) learning means that unions can learn from the past and current changes and diffuse that knowledge internally. This will help them to anticipate future changes and to develop innovate strategies (Lévesque and Murray 2010, 341–345).

Brinkmann et al. (2008) as well as Schmalz and Dörre (2014) incorporate some of the capabilities proposed by the authors of the two approaches presented in this section into their power resources theory. Due to their centrality in changing environments such as marketizing healthcare sectors, capabilities are regarded separately from power resources. The main capabilities detected in the literature will be outlined in more detail in the following subsections.

2.4.3.1 Framing and identity

Framing is a concept also used in Frege and Kelly's (2003) model. Originally devised by Benford and Snow (2000), it describes how social movements and trade unions can articulate or "frame" problems in various ways. Actors use frames of reference that define and legitimize their action and advance an agenda. Framing is an active and dynamic process that entails agency and impacts the degree of mobilization of stakeholders (Benford and Snow 2000, 614; Lévesque and Murray 2013).

The perception of an ability to act and a belief in self-efficacy are crucial preconditions for the formation of social movements (Van Zomeren, Postmes, and Spears 2008) and presumably also of trade union collective action. As mentioned above, in this way, Gamson and Meyer (1996) not only regard the perception of agency as a precondition for action and success but also argue that an optimistic rhetoric of change and the belief that action can have an impact can create political opportunities. As such, an "unrealistic" *perception* of the possible can alter what *is* possible. This opportunity frame can then work similar to a self-fulfilling prophecy (Gamson and Meyer 1996 but also Diani 1996; Goodwin and Jasper 1999).

This belief in agency and a call to action can be present to different extents in differing types of framing. Actors can identify and evaluate problems (diagnostic framing), suggest solutions for them (prognostic framing), or by presenting possibilities or rationales for action, they can motivate stakeholders to become active (motivational framing) (Benford and Snow 2000, 615 ff.; Kuypers 2009). Motivational framing can target both the members of the organization or the wider public. One obstacle to mobilizing workers in the health sector is their special professional ethos. Especially, strike activities are considered as ethically objectionable since they supposedly put patients at risk (Chadwick and Thompson 2000). This issue can be overcome, according to some authors, if this ethos is politicized (Briskin 2012, 290 f.; Wolf 2015), or, in other words, when striking is defined not only as necessary to improve working conditions but also as a necessary action to improve care quality.

In this way, framing is also closely related to trade union's identity. Depending on their identity, a union or a social movement can be oriented more or less toward conflict, or toward cooperation (Hunt, Benford, and Snow 1994). Trade union's identities can be located in an area of tension of three distinct orientations: (1) a market-orientation in which unions focus on the regulation of wage labor, (2) a society-orientation in which unions contribute to the improvement of social security and cohesion, as well as (3) a class-orientation that aims for sociopolitical mobilization and promotion of class interests in a radical oppositional, anti-capitalist, and militant way (Hyman 2001). This impacts how unions perceive opportunities and threats (Hunt, Benford, and Snow 1994), and the choice of their strategies (Hyman 2001). Union's identities that are oriented toward society or class and a corresponding framing of the conflict can motivate workers and other stakeholders in society. In many cases, unions are driven by their members' interest in better pay, security, and professional autonomy. One way to increase the leverage a campaign has is by framing it as an issue that goes beyond the self-interest of workers, for instance as an issue of the quality of public services, protection of the environment, democracy, or human dignity (Frege et al. 2004; Lowell and Cornfield 2007; Tattersall 2009). A shift to a "beyond-the-workplace" framing can have a mobilizing effect on both, workers and public. It corresponds with workers in elderly care that do not attribute deteriorating working conditions to decisions of their employer but regard it as a political problem (Schroeder 2017). Moreover, this framing can mobilize the public and can facilitate working in coalitions with other stakeholders. Furthermore, not only the mobilization of new repertoires can reshape collective frames of reference but these new frames can also trigger new repertoires of action (Tarrow 2011).

Finally, it must be noted that studying framing is difficult since strategic frames that determine the target, timing, and tactics of a coherent strategy cannot be directly observed but must often be inferred (Ganz 2000, 1010).

2.4.3.2 *Leadership and organizational practices*

Another capability that fosters the adaptation of strategies to new contexts is a diverse leadership. Leadership, in this context, does not necessarily refer to single leaders or the formal leader of an organization, but rather to leaders, or teams of leaders, in a specific context or conflict. Leadership teams that consist of (1) insiders and outsiders that combine a diversity of experience and salient knowledge will be most successful to heuristically recontextualize this knowledge to devise new strategies and adapt to new situations through bricolage or analogy. (2) Furthermore, a leadership with strong ties to constituencies will possess salient information on how to best recruit members. A leadership with weak ties will in turn have good access to a variety of actors and ideas that facilitate new alliances and again facilitate innovating strategies. (3) Finally, a leadership with a diversity of collective action repertoires will be able to adapt to changing environments and help develop new effective strategies (Ganz 2000, 1014–1016).

Furthermore, a union with accountability structures that bring forth democratic or entrepreneurial leadership will yield greater strategic capacity than bureaucratic leadership. Democratic leaders will possess useful knowledge of constituencies and have enough political skills to be selected by them. Self-selected entrepreneurial leaders will possess skills and intrinsic motivations associated with creative work since becoming part of the leadership was due to their own initiative. Both types of leadership are supposed to be more creative and yield more strategic capacity than bureaucratically selected leaders (Ganz 2000, 1018).

Strategic flexibility can also be increased by certain organizational practices, such as deliberation, learning, and the mobilization of constituencies from multiple resources. (1) If an organization practices regular, open, and authoritative deliberation and membership participation in decisions, this will give leaders access to salient information, diverse points of view and ways of doing things, as well as an opportunity to learn. This will facilitate strategic innovation. It will also motivate members to participate in decisions and to implement and commit to what they decided upon (Ganz 2000, 1014 ff.). The process of deliberation necessitates horizontal and hierarchical connections within the union and good internal structures of communication. Internal solidarity and a cohesive identity will help mediate internally between contending interests (Lévesque and Murray 2010, 338, 2013). Extensive deliberation can, however, prolong decision processes and undermine efficiency (Voss 2010, 377 f.). Nevertheless, deliberative procedures appear to be of crucial importance especially in times of marketization, since it represents a change and changes are likely to create dissatisfaction that causes an increased desire among members to voice their concerns (Hirschman 1970). (2) Learning from the past and the diffusion of that learning will help in devising effective strategies as well. In this way, new ideas of organizational practices, procedures, policies and programs, innovations to enhance resources, processes for membership engagement, use of new technologies, and new methods of recruitment can be made accessible and promoted throughout the whole organization (Lévesque and Murray 2010, 344 f.). (3) A mobilization of a constituency from multiple resources will increase strategic flexibility as it grants an organization a greater room to maneuver (Ganz 2000, 1016–1019). However, with multiple constituencies, unions face the challenge of intermediating between contending interests and ensuring inner cohesion. A strong collective identity as presented earlier in this section and unity in purpose can help unions with this endeavor (Hyman 2001; Lévesque and Murray 2010, 336 ff.).

2.4.3.3 Networking

Finally, networks and collaboration with other civil society actors also extend unions' strategic capacity. Unions have different capabilities to build and sustain collaborative action, as well as to create networks with other unions and the community. They need to intermediate between contending interests since potential allies may be involved for different reasons, may have different backgrounds, hold conflicting values, pursue their own interests, and hold different kinds of repertoires of contention (Turner 2006; Lévesque and Murray 2010, 344). Networks and collaboration can extend unions' financial and human resources, help them connect to new groups of workers, complement their expertise, increase legitimacy of their demands, and facilitate mobilization of popular support (Frege et al. 2004, 139–141). Unions will be most likely to enter coalitions when associational and structural power is weak or in decline, when they expand their policies of interest representation, e.g. to international labor standards or environment protection, or when they have activists or leaders with experience in other social movements (Frege et al. 2004, 145–149). Unions with a class or society orientation are also more likely to seek coalitions (Hyman 2001; Turner and Hurd 2001). Furthermore, suitable coalition partners have to be available (Locke 1992; Gindin 2016), as well as political opportunities and multiple points of access to policy, as found especially in decentralized political systems (Frege et al. 2004, 150).

The strategies that can be chosen based on the recognition of political opportunity, given the local-level leeway, and effectively using resources and capabilities will be presented in the following section.

2.5 Strategies

Finally, this section deals with the dependent variable put under consideration in this study, namely the strategies that unions can choose to respond to marketization and subsequent understaffing. First, this section gives a short definition of "strategy". Second, it aims to systematize the variety of strategies that are available to unions in the health sector, in order to later classify strategies used by unions in the case studies as similar or distinct. Third, it explains in more detail the four main strategies emerging from the systematization.

2.5.1 Definition

"Strategy is how we turn what we have into what we need to get what we want" (Ganz 2009, 8). It is the link between the use of resources and the aims a union hopes to achieve, or the way in which resources are translated into power to achieve a certain outcome (Ganz 2000, 1010). Power in this context is best understood in Lukes' (1974) sense as a "power to", meaning an agent's ability to further their own interests or affect those of others, as opposed to "power over". It is about empowering workers and a union's capacity to "represent workers' interests, to regulate work and to effect social change" (Lévesque and Murray 2010, 335). To achieve a purpose with a strategy, unions do not only need to *have* resources but also need to recognize them (McAlevey 2016) and possess the capability or the resourcefulness to *deploy* them in an effective and efficient way (Ganz 2000; Lévesque and Murray 2010).

Ganz (2009) regards three elements as critical to deploying resources to their maximum effect: targeting, tactics, and timing. Resources are used in a targeted way when they are committed to outcomes that have been judged likely to move one closer to one's goal. Resources are deployed tactically if they do not only unfold their maximum power but also limit the value of the opponent's resources. Finally, depending on timing, the value of one's resources can vary, and there are moments that promise greater opportunity than others (Ganz 2009, 9).

Strategy is often understood as the result of business-style long-term strategic planning. As Gardner (1989, 53 f.) points out, this way of thinking about strategy is not suitable for unions. This, however, does not mean that union activity is ad hoc or totally reactive. Unions act in strategic ways even if it is not planned in a structured process. They develop strategies through debate and compromise, during and outside of official union meetings or through direct actions of officials or member groups in their spheres of influence (Boxall and Haynes 1997, 569). Moreover, strategy usually includes the notion of being designed to achieve a particular set of goals. However, union strategies are largely irrespective of the objective and can be better defined as "characteristic means by which a union attempts to implement policy and achieve its goals" (Gardner 1989, 55). These means are not necessarily explicitly selected, but rather they are the result of an unconscious but customary process of "accretion of experience" (ibid.). Since unions can pursue differing strategies despite similarities in environment, Gardner (1989, 68) furthermore stresses the element of choice rather than determinism in this concept. Strategy in this perspective is defined as a framework for critical and decisive choices about ends and means of a union (Child 1972).

Strategy in this study is understood as the means to achieve a purpose. Resources are deployed to attain an objective. Capabilities increase an effective and efficient use of these resources. Strategy is further understood in terms of strategic choice and not deterministically. Therefore, strategies can also be deliberately changed. Nevertheless, I acknowledge that critical choices are often made unconsciously and incrementally through processes of debate and compromise.

2.5.2 Initial systematization

Empirical research on trade unions in the public (healthcare) sector has shown that unions have a variety of strategies at hand that they can choose from in the course of marketization. Studies from Britain (Foster and Scott 1998), Canada (Jalette and Hebdon 2012), and Germany (Greer, Schulten, and Böhlke 2013) show that unions can mobilize members in demonstrations, strikes, and other actions, mobilize allies in politics and civil society, use legal levers, such as litigation or arbitration, or influence change in cooperation with decision-makers through proposing alternatives and/or through direct participation as comanagers. Finally, where marketization cannot be prevented, they can negotiate over effects.

To systematize the broad range of anti-marketization strategies, and to later compare strategies used by unions in the case studies, this section attempts to develop a simple scheme that helps classifying different strategies along two dimensions. As a very broad distinction that covers the main strategies used in practice, trade unions can either (1) pursue an influence-oriented and consensual strategy in interaction with their interlocutors or (2) a more adversarial strategy considering their members' concerns (Schmitter and Streeck 1999). Furthermore, they can (3) address workplace or (4) beyond-the-workplace issues (Heery, Healy, and Taylor 2004; Cunningham and James 2010). Workplace strategies focus on narrow economic concerns, such as securing jobs, wages, and working conditions. "Beyond-the-workplace" strategies take external sociopolitical issues into account (Foster and Scott 1998, 144). In many cases, unions are driven by their members' interest in better pay, security, and professional autonomy. One way to increase the leverage of a campaign is by framing it as an issue that goes beyond the self-interest of workers, for instance as an issue of the quality of public services, protection of the environment, democracy, or human dignity (Frege et al. 2004; Turner and Cornfield 2007; Tattersall 2009). Accordingly, trade unions can include allies from civil society or not, as part of their strategy.

The extent to which unions pursue membership-oriented or influence-oriented strategies and frame their issues in narrow workplace terms or wider sociopolitical terms can be explained with their resources, capabilities, and – when considering the choice aspect of strategy – particularly their identity. Unions that are oriented toward class will tend to choose membership-oriented strategies and use both workplace and beyond-the-workplace framings. Unions that are oriented toward society might use both influence- or membership-oriented strategies, but are likely to frame their issues in terms of wider societal issues. Unions with a market orientation will, in turn, be likely to focus on the workplace and pursue an influence-oriented strategy (Hyman 2001).

The distinction between membership- or influence-orientation and addressing workplace or societal issues yields four types of strategies: (1) cooperation with decision-makers in order to shape the process and moderate negative effects (Rehder 2006), (2) organization and activation of members (Voss and Sherman 2000), (3) mobilization and cooperation with allies (Turner and Hurd 2001; Fairbrother 2008), and (4) political action and/or lobbying (Culpepper 2002; Streeck and Hassel 2003, 348). In the following sections, these four main types of strategies will be fleshed out.

2.5.3 Four types of strategies

The four main types of anti-marketization strategies resulting from the systematization described in the above section will be portrayed in more detail in the following subsections. These strategies can probably be regarded as the most common strategies in Germany and England. However, these strategies are not exhaustive, they represent ideal types and often appear in mixed forms (See Table 2.1).

Table 2.1 Typology of trade union strategies

	Influence-oriented and consensual	Membership-oriented and adversarial
Workplace-orientation	Business unionism, advocacy, partnership, comanagement (market orientation)	Organizing (class orientation)
Beyond-the-workplace orientation	Political action/Lobbying (society orientation)	Social movement unionism (class and society orientation)

Source: Schmitter and Streeck (1999), Cunningham and James (2010), Heery et al. (2004), Hyman (2001), Voss and Sherman (2003), Fairbrother (2008), Rehder (2014), Turner and Hurd (2001), own presentation.

2.5.3.1 *Advocacy, partnership, and comanagement*

Advocacy, partnership, and comanagement strategies aim at regulation of employment relations and usually target typical workplace issues. Unions pursuing these strategies are typically market-oriented and in favor of cooperative relations with employers to increase their influence. Typically used methods are bargaining, effects bargaining, provision of expertise, and proposition of alternatives.

The basis of partnership and comanagement strategies is advocacy. A union that takes an advocacy approach seeks one-time wins or narrow policy changes. It will not substantially involve ordinary people, but count on professional staff, lawyers, pollsters, researchers, and communication firms to wage the battle. The main method used is backroom negotiations. Advocacy does not permanently alter the relations of power (McAlevey 2016, 9 f.).

In a broad sense, social partnership can be defined as a relationship between unions and employers which usually has a political agenda that includes shared objectives or mutual gains and is marked by a high degree of cooperation and trust (Ackers and Payne 1998; Kochan and Osterman 1994). Partnership consists of "formally structured, ongoing relations of cooperation between unions and employers" (Fichter and Greer. 2004, 71). This can happen between unions and employer associations at the national, regional, or sectoral level, or between workers and management on the firm level (ibid.). At the firm level, social partnership is also called comanagement and refers to close consultation with management with a minimum level of conflict (Rehder 2006, 228). Lastly, partnership requires sanctions in the case that one side unilaterally violates cooperation (Fichter and Greer 2004, 71 f.).

Partnership agreements can be differentiated according to the balance of power between the parties. They can be employer-dominant, meaning they reflect primarily the employer's interest and are less favorable to the workers' side. The opposite would be labor-parity, or, in other words, arrangements with a balance of power and more equal outcomes (Crouch 1992).

Partnership is not under all circumstances a promising strategy. Especially in a political environment that is generally hostile to the inclusion of unions, there is, as Heery, Kelly, and Waddington (2003) found for Britain, little reason to engage in partnership. A study comparing British banks and retail stores with and without partnership agreements found no significant link between partnership and increased density. In addition, across a range of other industries, there was no influence of partnership on wages, working hours, or holidays. Even though companies with employment security agreements were less likely to implement compulsory redundancies, they had no effect on the rate of job loss and levels of felt insecurity (Cully 1999, 81 f.). In the same way, Kelly (2004) showed for Britain that companies with partnership agreements did not produce better outcomes in wages or unionization rates; on the contrary, partnership firms in industries marked by employment decline even shed jobs at a faster rate than nonpartnership firms. Similarly, Stuart and Lucio (2002) used the example of the British

Manufacturing, Science, and Finance Union to show the inadequacy of firm-level partnerships. The management side still acted unilaterally while granting limited transparency. Subsequently, unions were excluded from decisions about investments, training, staff, and planning. Some partnership agreements even diluted union influence through collective bargaining by instating a process of joint consultation and problem solving (Marks et al. 1998, 220 ff.). Furthermore, partnership strategies are difficult to integrate with other, rather confrontational approaches (Fichter and Greer 2004, 77–79).

In Germany, partnership is a widespread and highly institutionalized approach (Turner 1998, 18 f.). At the political level, German unions have been fairly successful to address the needs of a changing workforce using a partnership approach (Behrens, Fichter, and Frege 2003). Fichter and Greer (2004, 81 f.) identify five topics of partnership at the political level that support trade union revitalization: the regulation of unemployment, job evaluation schemes, sectoral pension funds, temporary employment, and the creation of new jobs. Nevertheless, the participation of the national Alliance for Jobs (1998–2002) was criticized internally by unions due to its meagre accomplishments (Fichter and Greer 2004, 81–83) and also, during the 2008 financial and economic crisis, more far-reaching union goals were dismissed by government and employers despite union involvement in corporatist management (Dribbusch and Schulten 2011, 143).

At the German regional and local level, the partnership strategy has proven to be rarely effective at rejecting employers' neoliberal proposals due to diminishing government support for unions (Fichter and Greer 2004, 83). Rehder (2006) also identified deficits of legitimacy in German company pacts for employment and competitiveness. Traditionally, partnership or comanagement was legitimized by its favorable outcome for employees. After years of concession bargaining, comanagement can no longer draw legitimacy from its output. Works councils therefore increasingly used membership participation to increase input legitimacy and thus reoriented their strategy toward more basis-orientation (Rehder 2006, 240).

Fichter and Greer (2004, 72) identified three preconditions that must be fulfilled for partnership to be successful and to lead to revitalization. (1) It needs to be embedded in a strong institutional framework that stipulates strong involvement of the union or workers, (2) it must be integrated in a proactive strategy and be complementary to other union strategies, and (3) it must be part of a broadly appealing social agenda. Only under these conditions will unions noticeably increase their bargaining and political power, as well as membership density. Fichter and Greer (2004, 88) note that unions, especially in the UK, are rarely able to realize all three conditions.

2.5.3.2 Organizing

The main goal of organizing is to increase organizational power. It usually also targets workplace issues. This strategy is linked to a class-oriented union identity and a membership-oriented, more adversarial attitude. In a narrow understanding

(Dörre 2013), typical methods used are recruitment, protests, strikes, as well as other direct actions and legal remedies.

To understand organizing, it is worth reviewing McAlevey's distinction between mobilizing and organizing. In contrast to advocacy, mobilizing brings large numbers of people to the fight. The main tool is campaigning. However, the campaign is directed, manipulated, and controlled by professional staff who are the key agents. The main focus is volunteer activists who are already committed, who "dutifully show up at protests". It matters little who shows up or why. Activists have no real say in campaigns and lack the full mass of their coworkers or community behind them. The campaign usually sets an ambitious goal and declares a win even if enforcement provisions are weak or nonexisting (McAlevey 2016, 10). Organizing also aims at the masses, but targets ordinary people who were never involved in political action before. It evolves around specific instances of injustice and outrage, but the campaigns fit into a larger power-building strategy. Ordinary people steer the campaign and "organic leaders" recruit new people who were not previously involved. Therefore, face-to-face interactions are key. Settlements typically come from negotiations that involve large numbers of people who gain their power from withdrawing labor or cooperation (McAlevey 2016, 10).

Since the concepts of organizing and Social Movement Unionism are often not clearly distinguished from one another, it is also worth differentiating between these two concepts. In addition, the concept of organizing, especially in the German context, is ambiguous with respect to its term and concept (Dörre 2013), and implies a rather diffuse concept and set of instruments (Dribbusch 2007). In essence, organizing aims at member recruitment (Voss and Sherman 2000). It was first developed in the US American Justice-for-Janitors campaign by the Service Employees International Union (SEIU). It was marked by the special character of the work that was site-dependent, characterized by a sensitive relationship between the customer and the cleaning firm, and the fact that the customers of the cleaning firms were discredited through trade union action that received public attention. The forms of action also showed a considerable degree of militancy. Furthermore, whipsawing of employees in different cleaning firms was evaded by offering them collective agreements with lower standards to stay competitive with nonorganized firms. When these competitors were organized, the firm returned to their original collective agreement. Moreover, SEIU built coalitions with other civil society organizations (Rehder 2014, 247–249). In the German version of organizing, some scholars also regard coalition building as part of organizing (Dribbusch 2007). However, in a narrow sense, organizing does not include intensive coalition work, rather coalition work has only instrumental character in promoting membership recruitment (Dörre 2013). In this study, organizing will be understood in a narrow sense to allow for a better distinction of organizing and social movement unionism.

The adoption of organizing by the German system of employment relations is regarded critically. Unions in coordinated market economies usually use their instrumental power to secure influence (Visser 1995, 53). However, in times of liberalization, this channel of influence becomes weaker and encourages the adoption of new strategies such as organizing (Rehder 2014, 252 f.). The dual structure of representation, or, in other words, representation in the workplace through the works council and by the trade union, can be an obstacle to organizing in Germany. This is because the level of collective bargaining presumably deprives the workplace level of certain issues around which members could be mobilized (Frege 2000, 276). This dual structure is also thought to inhibit an accumulation of conflict, thus reducing the overall potential for conflict (Müller-Jentsch 1997, 195). Furthermore, organizing is regarded as bearing the risk of questioning established local structures and of putting strain on social partnership (Frege 2000; Prott 2013; Rehder 2014; Rehder 2008). However, the German metalworkers' union IG Metall and ver.di used organizing in pilot projects and their evaluations were mainly positively (Bremme, Fürniß, and Meinecke 2007; Wetzel 2013). Central elements of organizing were also used in the ver.di campaign against the discounter Lidl in Germany (Rehder 2014, 249–252). Nachtwey and Thiel (2014) also showed with their study of two organizing projects in the hospital sector that ver.di can successfully use elements of organizing, even though the increase in membership was not sustainable after the organizing projects had been completed. This was attributed to an insufficient adaptation of the concept to the dual structure of interest representation in Germany. Furthermore, unionists require strategic capacity to successfully use organizing. They need to recognize and use opportunity structures at the workplace, societal, and political level (Nachtwey and Wolf 2013).

2.5.3.3 Social movement unionism

The main goal of social movement unionism is an increase in societal power. It usually targets beyond-the-workplace issues. This strategy is linked to a class-oriented union identity and a membership-oriented, more adversarial attitude. Typical methods used are networking with actors from civil society and public campaigns.

Social movement unionism describes a strategy through which change is negotiated with the support of worker and community mobilization (Baccaro, Hamann, and Turner 2003; Frege and Kelly 2004; Greer, Schulten, and Böhlke 2013, 220). It was first developed in the Anglo-American context, but, as Greer (2008) has shown in his study of social movement unionism in the hospital sector in the beginning of the 2000s, ver.di is also not institutionally confined to traditional strategies. The unions' influence and conflict ability can be increased through strategic coalition building and networking. The strategy's core elements are: (1) a local focus, (2) the establishment of broad societal alliances, (3) a political framing that refers to social justice and change, (4) the use of new forms of collective action and member recruitment, as well as (5) an emancipatory political approach to mobilize workers on the ground (Bezuidenhout 2000; Voss and Sherman 2000, 51; Turner and Hurd 2001; Turner 2003; Voss and Sherman 2003; Lopez 2004; Fairbrother 2008). It emerges in places where workers are excluded from the central decision-making process (Fairbrother 2008, 216). Social movement unionism embraces emancipatory politics, questions prevailing social formations, frames demands politically, and formulates transformative visions (Johnston 1994; Gindin 1995; Waterman 2001; Scipes 2003). This strategy necessitates a class-oriented union identity (Fairbrother 2008) and, of course, the presence of potential allies (Gindin 2016). Unions' networks can differ strongly between regions. Some may have dense networks of actors who work closely together to resolve industrial conflicts and advocate improvements; others may be confronted with a relatively demobilized civil society (Locke 1992).

In this context, McAlevey's reflections on the relationship between workers and their community appear worth considering. She suggests not viewing workers one-dimensionally as just workers but also as people who live in a community. They are understood as class actors in their communities. Power can be derived from systematically bringing their pre-existing community networks into their workplace fights. This is what she calls "whole worker organizing". The author stresses that the question is not only "if 'the grassroots'—are engaged, but *how, why*, and *where* they are engaged" (McAlevey 2016, 58). Most scholars, however, rather imply coalitions with existing actors when theorizing social movement unionism.

Unions can enter different types of coalitions. Frege et al. (2004) distinguish between different types of coalitions on the basis of the union's relationship with its allies and with the state. Relations to allies can be of the (1) vanguard, (2) common cause, or (3) integrative type. (1) Vanguard coalitions are based on a subordinate role of the partner that offers solidarity and support for the union's objective on an unconditional basis. The objective is supported because of its progressive character or because it embodies a class interest. Coalitions of this type usually evolve around major trials of strength such as long and bitter industrial disputes. (2) Common cause coalitions are based on common interests. Coalition partners enter the coalition to advance their own distinct yet associated and complementary interests. This type of coalition often forms around public service restructuring. In (3) integrative coalitions, the union takes over the objective of a nonlabor organization and reflects the fact that unions are value-based organizations. This coalition may, for instance, be formed when activists from new social movements enter positions in unions. However, this support needs to be balanced against their own interests; therefore, it usually only materializes where it is not linked to high costs and only in the areas that are remote from core union interests (Frege et al. 2004, 141–144).

Each of these coalitions then can be distinguished with respect to its integration into state policymaking. (1) Coalitions of influence are coalitions with other insiders that are, like unions, continuous and formal organizations. In these coalitions, unions are accepted as legitimate representatives, and they have good access to and engage in dialogue with ministers and civil servants to refine public policy. (2) Coalitions of protest in turn seek to generate external pressure on the government. Coalition partners are loose-structured local organizations. The initiative for these coalitions may come from the union base rather than the center and may even be sanctioned by union leaders (Frege et al. 2004, 144–145).

There are different motivations for unions to enter coalitions. Unions have usually sought coalitions to secure their traditional objectives. (1) In Britain, coalitions first appeared during public sector restructuring to moderate this development and protect jobs and incomes of members. These initiatives were driven by political exclusion under the Conservative government. Thus, unions will turn to coalitions when other power resources are weak. (2) Another incentive for coalitions are shared objectives. This is the case with work-related interests that extend beyond the employment relationship, for instance in cases of discrimination based on race or gender. (3) A third motivation is the import of social movement methods and styles of campaigning (Heery et al. 2003, 87 f.).

Not all coalitions will be successful. Gindin (2016) argues that debates of social movement unionism often underrate internal union problems, as well as weaknesses of social movements. Also Heery et al. (2003, 92) found limited effects of links with social movements for union revitalization. Tattersall (2013) identified conditions under which coalition unionism will yield success, such as social change, organizational development, and union renewal. First, based on her international comparative study of coalition success in the field of education, health, and living wages, she concludes that "less is more". Coalitions with fewer organizations will be stronger since it will be easier to build them, make decisions, and share resources. Furthermore, a coalition's success will depend on the leaders' ability to mediate between organizations and to develop a campaign strategy. Moreover, the success will depend on goals that combine organizational and public interests, and take into account electoral politics. Finally, Tattersall notes that the role of the individual is traditionally underestimated and should receive more attention.

2.5.3.4 Political action and lobbying

The main goal of lobbying is to influence political decisions. It usually targets employment issues. This strategy is linked to a market-oriented union identity and an influence-oriented, more cooperative attitude. Typical methods used are networking with decision-makers and public campaigns.

In most European welfare states, both trade unions and governments have an interest in including trade unions in the social policy governance. Trade unions can influence social policies by the electoral channel and by using veto points. They have an interest in negotiating reforms to avoid more severe welfare state retrenchment. Their involvement ranges from being party to social pacts and institutionalized consultation to informal agreements. Trade unions are most influential when the state devolves self-administrative functions that involve their social partners (Ebbinghaus 2011, 315).

In times of positive economic prospects, centralized trade unions in particular can offer governments wage moderation in exchange for favorable social policies and improved institutional conditions. In the past, unions were often unable to engage in the so-called "neo-corporatist political exchange" (Headey 1970; Schmitter 1977; Lehmbruch 1984), as they could not discipline their members and deliver wage moderation in exchange for political concessions by the government. Furthermore, engaging in political exchange bears the risk of member opposition and militancy, as well as member demotivation (Streeck and Hassel 2003, 344 f.).

Traditionally, based on common origins in the context of the labor movement, unions secured political influence through their close relationship to left or center-left political parties. However, only if unions can credibly threaten to shift their support and the votes of their members to a competing party can they increase their political clout. This ability seems to have declined since the beginning of the 2000s in both Germany and Britain (Streeck and Hassel 2003, 336, 345 f.).

Moreover, unions are included in governance structures. Through public institutions of functional representation such as social security funds or boards of quasi-public agencies they can influence the implementation of public policies. They usually have constitutional rights to advise the government or to be heard on current legislation (Streeck and Hassel 2003, 337). Nevertheless, the political power derived from this seems difficult to estimate as its key elements remain regulated by law (Rothstein 1992; Ebbinghaus 2002).

Informal inclusion of trade unions in policymaking has become increasingly important. Policymakers draw on concerned parties' expertise and cooperation to increase legitimacy. Given that their ties to social democratic parties have weakened, and functional representation tends to be pre-empted by state intervention and legislation, trade unions depend increasingly on classical lobbying. In this way, their opportunities have become similar to any other interest group (Culpepper 2002; Streeck and Hassel 2003, 348).

2.5.3.5 Other strategies, mixed forms, and strategic flexibility

The four main strategies in marketization conflicts presented above are, of course, not exhaustive and often appear in mixed forms. Strategies can be combined, for instance in the so-called "Konfliktpartnerschaft" (conflict partnership), in which unions sustain good relations with the management while strategically using conflict and pressure through worker mobilization to expand existing channels of influence (Müller-Jentsch 1999); or in the so-called comprehensive campaigning, which combines industrial, organizational, community, and political activities (Kaine and Rawling 2010). Apart from the presented strategies, unions also have a wide range of legal and legislative levers as Benz (2005) shows in her study of US organizing campaigns or Jalette and Hebdon (2012) show for public sector privatizations. Finally, unions can also choose to stay inactive (Jalette and Hebdon 2012; Greer, Schulten, and Böhlke 2013).

Last, but not least, it should be noted that unions are learning organizations and are not confined to bureaucratic conservatism, and they are able to deploy new or other strategies than previously. Unions can change their organization and established modes of action through "localized political crisis resulting in new leadership, the presence of leaders with activist experience outside the labour movement who interpret the decline of labour power as a mandate for change, and the influence of the international union in favour of innovation" (Voss and Sherman 2000, 341). In this way, Rehder (2014, 253) observed a shift from traditional corporatism to campaigning among German unions. Profound organizational change in unions will also entail a new relation between trade union officials and members (Lévesque, Murray, and Queux 2005). Especially in times of declining institutional power, strengthening organizational power appears crucial for trade union revitalization (Schmalz and Dörre 2014, 220 f.).

It has been argued above that resources and capabilities can be regarded as dynamic; they can – at least to a certain degree – be deliberately built, activated, and developed. Based on this assumption, unions are regarded as actors that can devise new strategies, combine different strategies, and change strategic orientations.

Note

1. It is worth noting that the authors explicitly distinguish their concept of capabilities from the more philosophical capabilities approach in the works of Sen (1992) and Nussbaum (2006) to avoid confusion (Lévesque and Murray 2010, 341).

References

Ackers, Peter, and Jonathan Payne. 1998. British Trade Unions and Social Partnership: Rhetoric, Reality and Strategy. *International Journal of Human Resource Management* no. 9 (3):529–550.

Baccaro, Lucio, and Chris Howell. 2011. A Common Neoliberal Trajectory: The Transformation of Industrial Relations in Advanced Capitalism. *Politics & Society* no. 39 (4):521–563.

Baccaro, Lucio, Kerstin Hamann, and Lowell Turner. 2003. The Politics of Labour Movement Revitalization: The Need for a Revitalized Perspective. *European Journal of Industrial Relations* no. 9 (1):119–133.

Bach, Stephen, and Lorenzo Bordogna. 2011. Varieties of New Public Management or Alternative Models? The Reform of Public Service Employment Relations in Industrialized Democracies. *International Journal of Human Resource Management* no. 22 (11):2349–2366.

Bambra, Clare. 2005. Worlds of Welfare and the Health Care Discrepancy. *Social Policy and Society* no. 4 (1):31–41.

Behrens, Martin, Kerstin Hamann, and Richard Hurd. 2004. Conceptualizing Labor Union Revitalization. In *Varieties of Unionism: Strategies for Union Revitalization in a Globalizing Economy*, edited by Carola Frege and John Kelly, 11–30. Oxford/New York: Oxford University Press.

Behrens, Martin, Michael Fichter, and Carola M Frege. 2003. Unions in Germany: Regaining the Initiative? *European Journal of Industrial Relations* no. 9 (1):25–42.

Behrens, Martin, Richard W. Hurd, and Jeremy Waddington. 2004. How Does Restructuring Contribute to Union Revitalization? In *Varieties of Unionism: Strategies for Union Revitalization in a Globalizing Economy*, edited by Carola Frege and John Kelly, 117–136. Oxford/New York: Oxford University Press.

Benassi, Chiara, Virginia Doellgast, and Katja Sarmiento-Mirwaldt. 2016. Institutions and Inequality in Liberalizing Markets: Explaining Different Trajectories of Institutional Change in Social Europe. *Politics & Society* no. 44 (11):117–142.

Benford, Robert D., and David A. Snow. 2000. Framing Processes and Social Movements: An Overview Assessment. *Annual Review of Sociology* no. 26 (1):611–639.

Bezuidenhout, Andries. 2000. Towards Global Social Movement Unionism? Trade Union Responses to Globalization in South Africa. http://www.ilo.org/inst.

Bordogna, Lorenzo. 2008. Moral Hazard, Transaction Costs and the Reform of Public Service Employment Relations. *European Journal of Industrial Relations* no. 14 (4):381–400.

Boxall, Peter, and Peter Haynes. 1997. Strategy and Trade Union Effectiveness in a Neo-Liberal Environment. *British Journal of Industrial Relations* no. 35 (4):567–591.

Bremme, Peter, Ulrike Fürniß, and Ulrich Meinecke. 2007. *Never Work Alone: Organizing – Ein Zukunftsmodell für Gewerkschaften*. Hamburg: VSA Verlag.

Brinkmann, Ulrich, Hae-Lin Choi, Klaus Dörre, Hajo Holst, Serhat Karakayali, and Catharina Schmalstieg. 2008. *Strategic Unionism: Aus der Krise zur Erneuerung? Umrisse eines Forschungsprogramms*. Wiesbaden: VS Verlag für Sozialwissenschaften.

Brinkmann, Ulrich, and Oliver Nachtwey. 2010. Krise und strategische Neuorientierung der Gewerkschaften. *Aus Politik und Zeitgeschichte* no. 60:21–29.

Briskin, Linda. 2012. Resistance, Mobilization and Militancy: Nurses on Strike. *Nursing Inquiry* no. 19 (4):285–296.

Chadwick, Ruth, and Alison Thompson. 2000. Professional Ethics and Labor Disputes: Medicine and Nursing in the United Kingdom. *Cambridge Quarterly of Healthcare Ethics* no. 9:483–497.

Child, John. 1972. Organizational Structure, Environment and Performance: The Role of Strategic Choice. *Sociology* no. 6 (3):1–22.

Chun, Jennifer Jihye. 2009. *Organizing at the Margins: The Symbolic Politics of Labor in South Korea and the United States*. Ithaca: ILR Press.

Crouch, Colin. 1992. The Fate of Articulated Industrial Relations Systems: A Stock-Taking after the 'Neo-Liberal' Decade. In *The Future of Labour Movements*, edited by Marino Regini, 169–187. London: SAGE.

Cully, Mark. 1999. *Britain at Work: As Depicted by the 1998 Workplace Employee Relations Survey*. London: Routledge.

Culpepper, Pepper D. 2002. Powering, Puzzling, and 'Pacting': The Informational Logic of Negotiated Reforms. *Journal of European Public Policy* no. 9 (5):774–790.

Culpepper, Pepper D. 2010. *Quiet Politics and Business Power: Corporate Control in Europe and Japan*. Cambridge University Press. Cambridge.

Cunningham, Ian, and Philip James. 2010. Strategies for Union Renewal in the Context of Public Sector Outsourcing. *Economic and Industrial Democracy* no. 31: 34–60.

Diani, Mario. 1996. Linking Mobilization Frames and Political Opportunities: Insights from Regional Populism in Italy. *American Sociological Review* no. 61 (December):1053–1069.

Doellgast, Virginia, and Ian Greer. 2007. Vertical Disintegration and the Disorganization of German Industrial Relations. *British Journal of Industrial Relations* no. 45 (1):55–76.

Dörre, Klaus. 2013. Organizing – Ein Konzept zur Erneuerung gewerkschaftlicher Organisationsmacht. https://heimatkunde.boell.de/2013/09/10/organizing-ein-konzept-zur-erneuerung-gewerkschaftlicher-organisationsmacht.

Dribbusch, Heiner. 2007. Das "Organizing-Modell" – Entwicklung, Varianten und Umsetzung. In *Never Work Alone: Organizing – Ein Zukunftsmodell für Gewerkschaften*, edited by Peter Bremme, Ulrike Fürniß and Ulrich Meinecke. Hamburg: VSA Verlag. 24–52.

Dribbusch, Heiner, and Thorsten Schulten. 2011. German Unions Facing Neo-Liberalism: Between Resistance and Accommodation. Gregor Gall, Adrian Wilkinson, Richard Hurd. *International Handbook of Labour Unions: Responses to Neo-Liberalism*, 143–166. Cheltenham: Edgar Elgar.

Ebbinghaus, Bernhard. 2002. Trade Unions' Changing Role: Membership Erosion, Organisational Reform, and Social Partnership in Europe. *Industrial Relations Journal* no. 33 (5):465–483.

Ebbinghaus, Bernhard. 2011. The Role of Trade Unions in European Pension Reforms: From 'Old' to 'New' Politics? *European Journal of Industrial Relations* no. 17 (4):315–331.

Fairbrother, Peter. 2008. Social Movement Unionism or Trade Unions as Social Movements. *Employee Responsibilities and Rights Journal* no. 20 (3):213–220.

Fichter, Michael, and Ian Greer. 2004. Analysing Social Partnership: A Tool of Union Revitalization? In *Varieties of Unionism: Strategies for Union Revitalization in a Globalizing Economy*, edited by Carola Frege and John Kelly. 71–92. New York, NY: Oxford University Press.

Foster, Deborah, and Peter Scott. 1998. Conceptualising Union Responses to Contracting Out Municipal Services, 1979–97. *Industrial Relations Journal* no. 29 (2):137–150.

Frege, Carola. 2000. Gewerkschaftsreformen in den USA. Eine kritische Analyse des 'Organisierungsmodells'. *Industrielle Beziehungen* no. 7 (3):260–280.

Frege, Carola, Edmund Heery, and Lowell Turner. 2004. The New Solidarity? Trade Union Coalition-Building in Five Countries. In *Varieties of Unionism: Strategies for Union Revitalization in a Globalizing Economy*, edited by Carola Frege and John Kelly. Oxford/New York: Oxford University Press.

Frege, Carola, and John Kelly. 2003. Union Revitalization Strategies in Comparative Perspective. *European Journal of Industrial Relations* no. 9 (7):7–24.

Frege, Carola, and John Kelly. 2004. Union Strategies in Comparative Context. In *Varieties of Unionism: Strategies for Union Revitalization in a Globalizing Economy*, edited by Carola Frege and John Kelly, 31–44. Oxford: Oxford University Press.

Galetto, Manuela, Paul Marginson, and Catherine Spieser. 2014. Collective Bargaining and Reforms to Hospital Healthcare Provision: A Comparison of the UK, Italy and France. *European Journal of Industrial Relations* no. 20 (2):131–147.

Gamson, William A., and Davis S. Meyer. 1996. 12 - Framing Political Opportunity. In *Comparative Perspectives on Social Movements: Political Opportunities, Mobilizing Structures, and Cultural Framings*, edited by Dough McAdam, John D. McCarthy and Mayer N. Zald, 275–290. Cambridge: Cambridge University Press.

Ganz, Marshall. 2000. Resources and Resourcefulness: Strategic Capacity in the Unionization of Californian Agriculture, 1959–1966. *The American Journal of Sociology* no. 105:1003–1062.

Ganz, Marshall. 2009. *Why David Sometimes Wins: Leadership, Organization, and Strategy in the California Farm Worker Movement*. Oxford: Oxford University Press.

Gardner, Margarete. 1989. Union Strategy: A Gap in Union Theory. In *Australian Unions: An Industrial Relations Perspective*, edited by Bill Ford and David Plowman, 49–72. Melbourne: Macmillan Education.

Gindin, Sam. 1995. *The Canadian Auto Workers: The Birth and Transformation of a Union*. Toronto: James Lorimer.

Gindin, Sam. 2016. Beyond Social Movement Unionism. *Jacobin*. https://www.jacobinmag.com/2016/08/beyond-social-movement-unionism/.

Glyn, A. 2006. *Capitalism Unleashed: Finance Globalization and Welfare*. Oxford: Oxford University Press.

Goodwin, Jeff, and James M. Jasper. 1999. Caught in a Winding, Snarling Vine the Structural Bias of Political Process Theory. *Sociological Forum* no. 14 (1):27–54.

Greer, Ian. 2008. Social Movement Unionism and Social Partnership in Germany: The Case of Hamburg's Hospitals. *Industrial Relations* no. 47 (4):602–624.

Greer, Ian, Thorsten Schulten, and Nils Böhlke. 2013. How Does Market Making Affect Industrial Relations? Evidence from Eight German Hospitals. *British Journal of Industrial Relations* no. 51 (2):215–239.

Greer, Ian, and Virginia Doellgast. 2017. Marketization, Inequality, and Institutional Change: Toward a New Framework for Comparative Employment Relations. *Journal of Industrial Relations* no. 59 (2):192–208.

Hall, Peter, and Daniel Gingerich. 2009. Varieties of Capitalism and Institutional Complementarities in the Political Economy. *British Journal of Political Science* no. 39:449–482.

Hall, Peter A., and David Soskice. 2001. An Introduction to Varieties of Capitalism. In *Varieties of Capitalism. The Institutional Foundations of Comparative Advantage*, edited by Peter A. Hall and David Soskice, 1–71. New York, NY: Oxford University Press.

Hassel, Anke. 1999. The Erosion of the German System of Industrial Relations. *British Journal of Industrial Relations* no. 37 (3):483–505.

Hassel, Anke. 2014. The Paradox of Liberalization – Understanding Dualism and the Recovery of the German Political Economy. *British Journal of Industrial Relations* no. 52 (1):57–81.

Hauptmeier, Marco. 2012. Institutions Are What Actors Make of Them – The Changing Construction of Firm-Level Employment Relations in Spain. *British Journal of Industrial Relations* no. 50 (4):737–759.

Headey, Bruce W. 1970. Trade Unions and National Wages Policies. *The Journal of Politics* no. 32 (2):407–439.

Heery, Edmund, Geraldine Healy, and Phil Taylor. 2004. Representation at Work: Themes and Issues. In *The Future of Worker Representation*, edited by Geraldine Healy, Edmund Heery, Phil Taylor and William Brown, 1–36. Basingstoke, NY: Palgrave Macmillan.

Heery, Edmund, John Kelly, and Jeremy Waddington. 2003. Union Revitalization in Britain. *European Journal of Industrial Relations* no. 9 (1):79–97.

Hirschman, Albert O. 1970. *Exit, Voice, and Loyalty: Responses to Decline in Firms, Organizations, and States*. Cambridge, MA: Harvard University Press.

Howell, Chris. 2006. Varieties of Capitalism: And Then There Was One?. *Comparative Politics* no. 36 (1):103–124.

Hunt, Scott A., Robert D. Benford, and David A. Snow. 1994. Identity Fields: Framing Processes and the Social Construction of Movement Identities. In *New Social Movements: From Ideology to Identity*, edited by Enrique Laraña, Hank Johnston and Joseph R. Gusfield, 185–208. Philadelphia: Temple University Press.

Hyman, Richard. 2001. *Understanding European Trade Unionism*. London: SAGE.

Jalette, Patrice, and Robert Hebdon. 2012. Unions and Privatization: Opening the "Black Box". *Industrial & Labor Relations Review* no. 65 (1):17–35.

Johnston, Paul. 1994. *Success While Others Fail: Social Movement Unionism and the Public Workplace*. Ithaca, NY: ILR Press.

Kaine, Sarah, and Michael Rawling. 2010. 'Comprehensive Campaigning' in the NSW Transport Industry: Bridging the Divide between Regulation and Union Organizing. *Journal of Industrial Relations* no. 52 (2):183–200.

Katz, Harry C., and Owen Darbishire. 2000. *Converging Divergences: Worldwide Changes in Employment Systems*. Ithaca/New York: ILR Press.

Kelly, John. 2004. Social Partnership Agreements in Britain: Labor Cooperation and Compliance. *Industrial Relations* no. 43 (1):267–292.

Kochan, Thomas, and Paul Osterman. 1994. *The Mutual Gains Enterprise: Forging a Winning Partnership among Labor, Management and Government*. Boston, MA: Harvard Business School Press.

Kuypers, Jim A. 2009. Framing Analysis. In *Rhetorical Criticism: Perspectives in Action*, edited by Jim A. Kuypers, 181–204. Lanham and Plymouth: Lexington Books.

Lehmbruch, Gerhard. 1984. Interorganisatorische Verflechtungen im Neokorporatismus. In *Politische Willensbildung und Interessenvermittlung*, edited by Jürgen W. Falter, Christian Fenner, Michael Th.Greven, 467–482. Opladen: Westdeutscher Verlag.

Lévesque, Christian, and Gregor Murray. 2010. Understanding Union Power: Resources and Capabilities for Renewing Union Capacity. *Transfer: European Review of Labour and Research* no. 16 (3):333–350.

Lévesque, Christian, and Gregor Murray. 2013. Renewing Union Narrative Resources: How Union Capabilities Make a Difference. *British Journal of Industrial Relations* no. 51:777–796.

Lévesque, Christian, Gregor Murray, and Stéphane Le Queux. 2005. Union Disaffection and Social Identity: Democracy as a Source of Union Revitalization. *Work and Occupations* no. 32 (4):400–422.

Locke, Richard M. 1992. The Demise of the National Union in Italy: Lessons for Comparative Industrial Relations Theory. *Industrial & Labor Relations Review* no. 45 (2):229–249.

Lopez, Steven Henry. 2004. *Reorganizing the Rust Belt: An Inside Study of the American Labor Movement*. Berkeley, California: University of California Press.

Lowell, Daniel B., and Cornfield. 2007. *Labor in the New Urban Battlegrounds: Local Solidarity in a Global Economy*. Ithaca: Cornell University Press.

Lukes, Steven. 1974. *Power: A Radical View*. London: MacMillan.

Mares, I. 2000. Strategic Alliances and Social Policy Reform: Unemployment Insurance in Comparative Perspective. *Politics & Society* no. 28 (2):223–244.

Marks, Abigail, Patricia Findlay, James Hine, Paul Thompson, and Alan McKinlay. 1998. The Politics of Partnership? Innovation in Employment Relations in the Scottish Spirits Industry. *British Journal of Industrial Relations* no. 36 (2):209–226.

McAlevey, Jane F. 2016. *No Shortcuts: Organizing for Power in the New Gilded Age*. Oxford University Press. Newyork.

Müller-Jentsch, Walther. 1997. *Soziologie der industriellen Beziehungen: Eine Einführung*. 2. Aufl. Frankfurt am Main/New York: Campus.

Müller-Jentsch, Walther. 1999. *Konfliktpartnerschaft: Akteure und Institutionen der industriellen Beziehungen*. München: Rainer Hampp Verlag.

Nachtwey, Oliver, and Luigi Wolf. 2013. Strategisches Handlungsvermögen und Gewerkschaftliche Erneuerung im deutschen Modell industrieller Beziehungen. In *Comeback der Gewerkschaften? Machtressourcen, Innovative Praktiken, Internationale Perspektiven*, edited by Stefan Schmalz and Klaus Dörre, 104–123. Frankfurt am Main/ New York: Campus.

Nachtwey, Oliver, and Marcel Thiel. 2014. Chancen und Probleme Pfadabhängiger Revitalisierung. Gewerkschaftliches Organizing im Krankenhauswesen. *Industrielle Beziehungen* no. 21 (3): 257–276.

Nussbaum, Martha. 2006. *Frontiers of Justice: Disability, Nationality, Species Membership*. Cambridge, MA: The Belknap Press of Harvard University Press.

Offe, Claus, and Helmut Wiesenthal. 1980. Two Logics of Collective Action: Theoretical Notes on Social Class and Organizational Form. *Political Power and Social Theory* no. 1:67–115.

Palier, Bruno, and Kathleen Thelen. 2010. Institutionalizing Dualism: Complementarities and Change in France and Germany. *Politics & Society* no. 38 (1):119–148.

Prott, Jürgen. 2013. Organising als riskante gewerkschaftliche Erneuerungsstrategie. In *Organisieren am Konflikt: Tarifauseinandersetzung und Mitgliederentwicklung im Dienstleistungssektor*, edited by Andrea Kocsis, Gabriele Sterkel and Jörg Wiedemuth, 235–254. Hamburg: VSA.

Rehder, Britta. 2006. Legitimitätsdefizite des Co-Managements: Betriebliche Bündnisse für Arbeit als Konfliktfeld zwsichen Arbeitnehmern und betrieblicher Interessenvertretung. *Zeitschrift für Soziologie* no. 35 (3):228–242.

Rehder, Britta. 2008. Revitalisierung der Gewerkschaften? Die Grundlagen amerikanischer Organisierungserfolge und ihre Übertragbarkeit auf deutsche Verhältnisse. *Berliner Journal für Soziologie* no. 18 (3):342–456.

Rehder, Britta. 2014. Vom Korporatismus zur Kampagne? Organizing als Strategie der gewerkschaftlichen Erneuerung. In *Handbuch Gewerkschaften in Deutschland*, edited by Wolfgang Schroeder, 241–264. Wiesbaden: Springer Fachmedien.

Rothstein, Bo. 1992. Labor-Market Institutions and Working-Class Strength. In *Structuring Politics: Historical Institutionalism in Comparative Analysis*, edited by Sven Steinmo, Kathleen Thelen and Frank Longstreth, 33–56. New York, NY: Cambridge University Press.

Schmalz, Stefan, and Klaus Dörre. 2014. Der Machtressourcenansatz: Ein Instrument zur Analyse gewerkschaftlichen Handlungsvermögens. *Industrielle Beziehungen* no. 21 (3):217–237.

Schmitter, Philippe C. 1977. Modes of Interest Intermediation and Models of Societal Change in Western Europe. *Comparative Political Studies* no. 10 (1):7–38.

Schmitter, Philippe C., and Wolfgang Streeck. 1999. The Organization of Business Interests – Studying the Associative Action of Business in Advanced Industrial Societies. *MPIfG Discussion Paper* no. 99 (1).

Schroeder, Wolfgang. 2017. *Interessenvertretung in der Altenpflege: Zwischen Staatszentrierung und Selbstorganisation.* Wiesbaden: Springer-Verlag.

Scipes, Kim. 2003. Understanding the New Labor Movements in the "Third World": The Emergence of Social Movement Unionism, a New Type of Trade Unionism. http://www.labournet.de/diskussion/gewerkschaft/smu/The_New_Unions_Crit_Soc. htm#_edn1.

Sen, Amartya. 1992. *Inequality Reexamined*. New York: Oxford University Press.

Silver, Beverly J. 2003. *Forces of Labor: Workers' Movements and Globalization Since 1870*. Cambridge: Cambridge University Press.

Streeck, Wolfgang. 2009. *Re-Forming Capitalism: Institutional Change in the German Political Economy*. Oxford: Oxford University Press.

Streeck, Wolfgang, and Anke Hassel. 2003. Trade Unions as Political Actors. In *International Handbook of Trade Unions*, edited by John T. Addison and Claus Schnabel, 335–365. Cheltenham/Massachusetts: Edward Elgar.

Streeck, Wolfgang, and Kathleen Thelen. 2005. *Beyond Continuity: Institutional Change in Advanced Political Economies*. New York: Oxford University Press.

Stuart, Mark, and Miguel Martínez Lucio. 2002. Social Partnership and the Mutual Gains Organization: Remaking Involvement and Trust at the British Workplace. *Economic and Industrial Democracy* no. 23 (2):177–200.

Tarrow, Sidney G. 2011. *Power in Movement: Social Movements and Contentious Politics*. New York, NY: Cambridge University Press.

Tattersall, Amanda. 2009. A Little Help from Our Friends: Exploring and Understanding When Labor-Community Coalitions Are Likely to Form. *Labor Studies Journal* no. 34 (4):485–506.

Tattersall, Amanda. 2013. *Power in Coalition: Strategies for Strong Unions and Social Change*. Ithaca, NY: Cornell University Press.

Turner, Lowell. 1998. *Fighting for Partnership: Labor and Politics in Unified Germany*. Ithaca, NY: ILR Press.

Turner, Lowell. 2003. Reviving the Labor Movement: A Comparative Perspective. *Research in the Sociology of Work* no. 11:23–58.

Turner, Lowell. 2006. Globalization and the Logic of Participation: Unions and the Politics of Coalition Building. *Journal of Industrial Relations* no. 48:83–97.

Turner, Lowell, and Richard W. Hurd. 2001. Building Social Movement Unionism. The Transformation of the American Labor Movement. In *Rekindling the Movement. Labor's Quest for Relevance in the 21st Century*, edited by Lowell Turner, Harry C. Katz and Richard W. Hurd, 9–26. Ithaca, NY: ILR Press.

Van Zomeren, Martijn, Tom Postmes, and Russell Spears. 2008. Toward an Integrative Social Identity Model of Collective Action: A Quantitative Research Synthesis of Three Socio-Psychological Perspectives. *Psychological Bulletin* no. 4/2008:504–535.

Visser, Jelle. 1995. Trade Unions from a Comparative Perspective. In *Comparative Industrial and Employment Relations*, edited by Joris van Ruysseveldt, Rien Huiskamp and Jacques van Hoof, 37–67. London: SAGE.

Voss, Kim. 2010. Democratic Dilemmas: Union Democracy and Union Renewal. *Transfer* no. 16 (3): 369–382.

Voss, Kim, and Rachel Sherman. 2000. Breaking the Iron Law of Oligarchy: Union Revitalization in the American Labor Movement. *American Journal of Sociology* no. 106 (2):303–349.

Voss, Kim, and Rachel Sherman. 2003. You Just Can't Do It Automatically: The Transition to Social Movement Unionism in the United States. In *Trade Unions in Renewal: A Comparative Study*, edited by Peter Fairbrother and Charlotte Yates, 51–77. London: Continuum.

Wagner, Ines. 2015. Rule Enactment in a Pan-European Labour Market: Transnational Posted Work in the German Construction Sector. *British Journal of Industrial Relations* no. 53 (4):692–710.

Waterman, Peter. 2001. Trade Union Internationalism in the Age of Seattle. In *Place, Space and the New Labour Internationalisms*, edited by Peter Waterman and Jane Wills, 8–32. Oxford: Blackwell.

Wetzel, Detlef. 2013. *Organizing: Die Veränderung der gewerkschaftlichen Praxis durch das Prinzip Beteiligung*. Hamburg: VSA Verlag.

Wolf, Luigi. 2015. Mehr von uns ist besser für alle: die Streiks an der Berliner Charité und ihre Bedeutung für die Aufwertung von Care-Arbeit. In *UMCARE: Gesundheit und Pflege neu organisieren*, edited by Barbara Fried and Hannah Schurian, 23–31. Berlin: Rosa-Luxemburg-Stiftung.

Wright, Erik O. 2000. Working Class Power, Capitalist Class Interests, and Class Compromise. *American Journal of Sociology* no. 105 (4):957–1002.

3 Handling the beginnings of marketization

Partnership approaches to corporatization

3.1 Introduction

Formal privatization or corporatization of hospitals is a form of marketization that is widely applied, but also widely neglected and under-researched due to a lack of available data (for a detailed account on formal privatization processes see Chapter 1). The transformation of hospitals' legal form from public to private is not highly politicized, since state ownership is maintained and it seems to have limited impact for employees and the quality of care. Its advantages, in turn, seem obvious: increased entrepreneurial freedom, easier access to capital markets, improved competitiveness and economic sustainability. However, corporatization is often the first step that facilitates the implementation of financial restrictions, as well as other forms of marketization, such as outsourcing of support and medical services or hospital sell-offs. These processes usually lead to competition on the costs of labor and thus work intensification and a deterioration of care quality (Obinger, Schmitt, and Traub 2016).

There is little research dealing with trade union responses specific to hospital corporatization. This might be due to a low political salience and subsequently relatively weak trade union responses to it, as well as due to its relatively small and containable effects on employees and employment relations. Corporatization is a form of marketization that seems to be particularly difficult for unions to oppose. Since hospitals remain in public ownership, it appears to be a "mild" form of marketization. It is a small step toward marketization, usually justified pragmatically, therefore more difficult to oppose than single profound and ideologically justified actions (Doellgast and Greer 2007; Givan and Bach 2007). As Kahancová and Szabó (2015) showed for the Hungarian and Slovenian hospital sector, corporatization does not automatically bring about institutional change in bargaining patterns – even though it is theoretically possible. Employers and unions remained committed to bargaining practices, wage levels and public collective agreement provisions, therefore securing the pre-corporatization status quo. Also in the NHS, with a single exception, corporatized trusts did not deviate from the nationally agreed Agenda for Change pay system, even though it would have been theoretically possible (Galetto, Marginson, and Spieser 2014). Consequently, as will be shown in Section 3.3, corporatization often appears to be a merely technical exercise. Thus, it deserves relatively little attention in the unions' publications and does not provoke strong union action. However, union action influences the effect of corporatization. As Kaminska and Kahancová (2017) showed in a study of Poland, Hungary, Czech Republic and Slovenia, the modes of regulation of sectoral employment and working conditions can differ considerably, despite comparable governmental policies. The differences that arise depend on the fragmentation of the union movement and their associational power, governments' susceptibility to trade union demands and employers' ability and willingness to cooperate with them.

Furthermore, corporatization can create financial pressures. Since wages can account for 60 to 85 per cent of total operating expenses (Schwartz 2001, 28), focusing on cost containment can lead to a deterioration of working conditions (Kühn and Klinke 2006; Marrs 2007). Furthermore, cost containment can also have a negative impact on care quality. This can be illustrated with evidence from Britain. To demonstrate their financial viability to qualify for the private legal form of a foundation trust, NHS trusts neglected the quality of their care. This came to the attention of the public through the Mid-Staffordshire scandal investigated in the Keogh Report in 2013. The report expressed significant concerns around inadequate staffing levels, nursing skill mix, and poor workforce planning, particularly out of hours. The author of the report, Sir Bruce Keogh, National Medical Director of the NHS England, attributed this to a distraction of foundation trusts by efficiency saving requirements:

> A number of the trusts have been undergoing mergers, restructures or applications for foundation trust status and many have needed to make significant cost savings. These issues may have diverted management time and attention from focusing on quality.
>
> (Keogh 2013, 29)

Furthermore, the increase in mergers observed between 2010 and 2015 was often motivated by the pursuit of foundation trust status and judged as not always being rational and not always taking into account the business case (Collins 2015). Thus, corporatization is not necessarily reasonable but can also set incentives that work to the detriment of care quality and working conditions.

Irrespective of its usual low political salience, corporatization is worth studying since it is usually a precondition for further forms of marketization. Moreover, the maintenance of the status quo in bargaining patterns, wages and working conditions does not happen automatically, but must be secured each time the corporatization process takes place and continuously. Therefore, unions have a reason to become active in corporatization processes. In addition, the restructuring process accompanying corporatization can potentially be used by the unions as an opportunity structure. As will be shown, corporatization can be used by the union to strengthen its role in partnership and to realize its own demands related to the hospital structure. However, the cases will confirm the conclusions of Fichter and Greer (2004), who argue that partnership strategies will only be successful if they meet the three preconditions of: (1) being embedded in a strong institutional framework that stipulates strong involvement of the union or workers, (2) being integrated in a proactive strategy and complementary to other union strategies, as well as (3) being part of a broadly appealing social agenda.

Given that the cases to be studied are situated in two most-different settings, it can be assumed that trade unions choose differing strategies in the corporatization process. However, they are confronted with the same form of marketization, which creates similar, relatively low pressures for unions. Corporatization was not highly politicized and had limited direct effects on the workforce in both countries. Therefore, trade unions in both countries are expected to pursue an influence-oriented, cooperative strategy. Nevertheless, their influence will depend on their endowment with power resources and on their capabilities.

In this chapter, I will give a brief overview of the two cases of corporatization in Germany and England. Subsequently, findings based on document analysis and semi-structured interviews will be presented. The chapter will end with a comparison of the two case studies and a conclusion.

3.2 Information on corporatization cases

The comparison of trade union strategies with regards to corporatization processes of large metropolitan hospitals is embedded in a most-different systems design. Cases in this chapter are defined as trade union strategies designed to prevent corporatization or mitigate its effects. Despite differing national institutional settings, unions pursued similar strategies of partnership in the course of corporatization (also see Chapter 1 for more details on the overall research design).

The first case, the municipal hospitals of Berlin, Vivantes, is the result of a merger of nine municipal hospitals in Berlin with about 5,471 beds, 14,714 staff, and an annual turnover of €1.02bn (2014) (Vivantes 2017). Vivantes was transformed into a limited-liability company (GmbH) in 2001 and was an early case of formal privatization. Most formal privatizations in Germany took place between 2002 and 2006 (ver.di Infodienst Krankenhäuser 2001–2016). From 2007, the share of public hospitals in private legal form remained stable at 18 per cent (Statistisches Bundesamt 2016). Therefore, the time frame of this case study differs from the case studies in the other empirical chapters. Compared to other cases of formal privatization studied in the document analysis, Vivantes represents a typical case, with its strategical orientation toward comanagement and relatively low political salience. The English case study examines the corporatization of the Guy's and St. Thomas' NHS Trust (GSTT). It is composed of two trusts in London with 15,000 staff and an annual turnover of £1.3bn (2015–2016) (Guy's and St. Thomas' NHS Foundation Trust 2016). The GSTT was transformed into a foundation trust in 2004 and thus also represents a relatively early case of formal privatization. The documents studied from UNISON show that foundation trust transformations were usually not politicized or accompanied by trade union opposition. In this sense, the GSTT represents a typical case too

(UNISON 1995–2004, 2004–2015). However, UNISON's GSTT Branch was evaluated as particularly active and competent, and was recommended for a case study by the UNISON London Regional Manager in Health.

Both cases occurred relatively early in comparison to other forms of marketization because corporatization usually comes first. Furthermore, the trend to corporatization is slowing down (see further below), and corporatization is further depoliticized due to a habituation effect.

Despite the comparable timing of corporatization, size, turnover, and metropolitan location of the hospital groups studied, UNISON and ver.di were acting in the most-different settings of liberal and coordinated market economies, as well as welfare, health, and employment relations systems (Esping-Andersen 1990; Hall and Soskice 2001; Böhm et al. 2013). Regardless of these differences, both trade unions pursued a partnership strategy.

The comparison is based on 16 interviews with trade unionists, management, a local politician, and a works council consultant (5 in England, 11 in Germany) that were conducted in 2015 and 2016 (quotes from interviews marked as "IP"), as well as a document analysis of the monthly published magazines "ver.di Infodienst Krankenhäuser" (IK) and the "UNISON InFocus" from 2001 to 2015 (for more information on data generation and analysis see Section 1.4.3).

3.3 Trade union responses to corporatization

This section will give an overview of general trends in trade union responses to corporatization and then present the empirical findings of the two case studies in more detail.

As mentioned above, the transformation of a hospital or trust into a private legal form while remaining in majority public ownership is one of the less contested forms of marketization, supposedly due to its low salience, high technicality, pragmatic justification, and incremental character.

This can be illustrated with findings from Germany, drawing on a document analysis of the "ver.di Infodienst Krankenhäuser". Out of 118 reported conflicts that dealt with marketization of the hospital sector (either formal, functional or material privatization, or containment of their effects) between 2001 and 2015, only 9 (8per cent) concerned formal privatization as a major issue and in another 8 cases (7per cent) it was a secondary issue (i.e., the main conflict concerned other forms of marketization). In the overwhelming majority of corporatization cases, trade unions engaged in comanagement. In three cases they remained quiescent.

However, in 2015, ver.di strongly opposed formal privatization of the municipal hospitals in Dresden that the Conservative municipal government was planning. This can be attributed to special local circumstances. Together with an alliance of Social Democrats, Greens and the Left, ver.di anticipated, based on experience in other cities, that formal privatization would lead to full privatization. The union initiated a referendum that was to decide on both formal and material privatization. Years earlier, ver.di had lobbied for rendering referenda legally binding in Saxony. A successful mobilization that was embedded in a wider political debate on profit-making in the hospital sector then led to a rejection of both the corporatization and the sell-off. Since then, Dresden has avoided all forms of privatization and all parties have successfully engaged in restructuring the hospitals in a sustainable way, which will make privatization less likely in the future (IP29, IP35, IP36; IK 03/2012). As mentioned above, this combination of adversarial social movement unionism and cooperative comanagement strategy represents an untypical case. As a business consultant who consults for works councils in hospital restructuring processes argued, employees and unions are not necessarily worse off in a company with limited liability if they succeed in negotiating comprehensive codetermination rights and strong transfer agreements. If there is a strong political will, also hospitals in *public* legal form can be sold. However, hospitals in public legal form cannot establish their own subsidiaries. This has to be done by the municipality or the state, which is more complex than for a hospital in private legal form (IP25: 54–60). This is probably why ver.di preferred engaging in comanagement and bargaining effects of corporatization rather than strict and confrontational opposition.

This tendency could be observed in England as well, even though corporatization there seemed even less contested than in Germany. Only 9 out of 348 articles (3per cent) related to marketization of the "UNISON InFocus" magazine dealt with transformations of trusts into foundation trusts. Half of them related to the general topic and the union's general position on foundation trusts and half of them concerned cases in which UNISON opposed specific transformations. In general, trade unionists in England clearly stated that they opposed foundation trusts: "UNISON opposed the proposal [Health and Social Care (Community Care and Standards) Act 2003] from the start" (IP09: 20). The union argued that it would create a two-tier health service, with finance being diverted to foundation trusts at the expense of other health sector organizations (IP05: 12–464, IP09: 20). Furthermore, they were concerned that trusts could get into financial difficulty because of the finance structures placed on foundation trusts that could impact staff conditions. Moreover, foundation trusts could have used their autonomy to set specific terms and conditions to the detriment of employees (IP09: 23 f., IP13: 6). Subsequently, Trade Union Congress (TUC) unions "mounted a vigorous campaign" (IP09: 1) against it. It included lobbying Members of Parliament and local councilors, protests addressed to the Secretary of State for Health, petitions, informing the public about the consequences of these changes through leaflets, and public meetings (IP05: 14–943, IP12: 5, IP09: 12, 23 f.). The campaign was run on both the national and subnational level and was eventually judged as "partly successful" (IP09: 8). Even though it did not prevent trusts from becoming foundation trusts, at least terms and conditions of staff were not affected. This was due to successful negotiations with the Labour Government over the introduction of a new national pay and grading structure in 2004, the Agenda for Change National Terms and Conditions of Employment (AfC),[1] which was not binding for foundation trusts, but they nevertheless adhered to it (IP09: 8, 27). Apart from one foundation trust in East Anglia, all foundation trusts applied the new

Agenda for Change National Terms and Conditions of Employment introduced in 2006 (IP09: 23 f.). This was attributed to strong local partnership structures (IP13: 6). However, there is an incentive for trusts to adhere to the AfC due to a staff shortage in the NHS (IP22: 4–69). The introduction of the AfC might have contributed to the depoliticization of corporatization since it moderated the most direct impact on workers, the change of terms and conditions.

In both case studies that will be outlined in the following sections, trade unions did not take a stance of blanket opposition. Ver.di and UNISON engaged mainly in partnership work to shape the restructuring process, however, with different degrees of influence.

3.3.1 Findings: England

The Guy's and St Thomas' NHS Trust (GSTT) was transformed into a foundation trust in 2004. The main driver was supposedly the government policy to turn all NHS trusts into foundation trusts – initially by 2008 – as stipulated in the Health and Social Care Act in 2003, as well as the increased financial and entrepreneurial freedoms that were associated with it and desirable for NHS trusts (Leys and Player 2011, 23). The local GSTT union officer quoted the possibilities of treating an increased share of private patients and of bargaining pay locally as a foundation trust as the reasons for the management's decision for transformation (IP22: 3–58). However, it is questionable if the latter can be regarded as a driving force of formal privatization since deviating from the national collective agreement was so far only used in practice by one foundation trust (Galetto, Marginson, and Spieser 2014).

3.3.1.1 Resources and capabilities

To secure participation in the process of transformation into a foundation trust, UNISON could draw on certain resources and capabilities. However, it barely used its power resources due to its market orientation and a lack in capabilities to recognize the opportunity to make its own suggestions, and to include its members.

UNISON's most used power resource was institutional, i.e., good access to management that it had built up over a period of 10 to 15 years despite limited personnel resources and a reliance on support from the regional and national union level (IP22: 9–62). The GSTT union secretary promoted good relations with the management through the persistent pursuit of a cooperative business unionism approach (IP22: 5–61). In comparison with other unions in the trust, UNISON had the closest relationship with management (IP22: 14–68, 8–62). There was also little competition for UNISON because it was the most visible and established union on the ground (IP22: 14–68, 8–62). In turn, associational power resources did not seem to have played a role in the GSTT case. The trade union secretary claimed that membership density was not important for his work. According to him, UNISON at the GSTT "already speak[s] on behalf of all staff" (IP22: 9–68) and their influence on management is so strong that they "[do] not need to use any leverage" (IP22: 9–68) such as trade union density. Members were also perceived as unwilling to engage in militant action such as strikes (IP22: 14–59). Allying with civil society actors, support of the public and access to media (societal power) were not mentioned during the interview; therefore, they did not appear as important resources for UNISON in the corporatization process (IP22: 8–65, 12–57). However, given the strong public support for the NHS in Britain (Halbwachs 1985), power could potentially have been drawn from this resource. In addition, given staff shortages in nursing (Kuehn 2007), UNISON could have exploited this structural power resource to their benefit.

The trade union representatives' framing of the trade union's role matched its clear reliance on its institutional power: "When it has to happen, I think that we as trade unions need to be a part of that process in order to make sure that the best can be made of a bad situation" (IP22: 9–52). The transformation as such was not questioned, and preventing it was not an option (IP22: 9–62). UNISON showed a business unionism identity by taking a pragmatic stance toward the issue and regarding the transformation process as an internal and administrative exercise (IP22: 8–65, 12–57). Their general self-concept resembled the role of a mediator as they describe themselves as "experts at getting people to talk to each other. […] Our real business is being a conduit for the information", through the means of reporting employees' opinions and expertise with respect to changes back to the management (IP22: 18–57).

3.3.1.2 Strategies

Coherent with its strong reliance on institutional power, its framing of the issue and union identity, UNISON focused on partnership and comanagement instead of organizing and mobilizing members. UNISON pursued a very cooperative partnership approach and managed to alter the relations with management. Throughout the 10 to 15 years of his activity as an activist and a representative, the UNISON GSTT secretary attained a seat on the trust board and the trust management executive.

> My vision was to build bridges because I figured that we are better off knowing what is happening rather than not. So, we created relationships and we got invited to meetings that we didn't have any right to be at.
>
> (IP22: 5–61)

Militancy was regarded as an inappropriate strategy at the local level: "There are two different levels, [the] local level and [the] national. When I talk about militancy, it can only be done nationally. Locally you have to work in partnership." (IP22: 10–51). Partnership, according to UNISON, required trustful relations, so militancy was unsuitable (IP22: 11–62). Furthermore, the branch secretary in GSTT believed that strikes had to be member-led, and since he perceived their members as unwilling to strike, this was not an option (IP22: 14–59).

Furthermore, in the GSTT trust, the transformation to a foundation trust and the introduction of the Agenda for Change coincided, thus fostering the partnership. As mentioned above, the AfC removed trade unions' fear and a potential point of contention that trusts could make use of their right to bargain local collective agreements. It also secured active participation of trade unionists in the process of re-evaluating pay and job profiles (IP22: 1–60, 2–68). The partnership approach was, according to the trade union representative, initially kept to the AfC, but it extended and developed into all areas of the business (IP22: 5–58). Furthermore, it was later laid down in a partnership agreement (IP22: 8–65). However, except for the re-evaluation process, the trade unionist interviewed described the agreement as "more of a paper exercise, so it was not meaningful" (IP22: 9–53). Notwithstanding, the partnership was considered very successful (IP22: 7–62). The way in which management and UNISON worked together was regarded as exemplary in UNISON and was spread as an example of good practice through joint presentations of the GSTT chief executive and trade union secretary (IP22: 8–62).

Membership interaction was widely restricted to servicing members and dealing with their individual work-related problems. In theory, the branch secretary was aware that "Our marketing strategy leads people to believe that we are no better than an insurance policy" and pleaded for more education for members about the necessity of trade unions and empowerment (IP22: 10–67, 12–52, 12–57), as well as bringing members into trade unionism (IP22: 14–59). However, members were not included in the transformation – presumably because it was not regarded as a contested issue, and involvement of the trade union representatives was deemed sufficient.

3.3.1.3 Outcome

The partnership with GSTT management that was established through years of cooperation, also through the Agenda for Change implementation, was evaluated as a success for the union (IP22: 7–62). UNISON did not regard the transformation as an issue in itself, and thus it did not formulate any demands in the process. Critical points on corporatization concerning, for instance, its impact on financial stability of the trust and care quality, could have been raised and could have been a reason for resistance, but were not. None of these were brought up by UNISON in GSTT in the process. This can probably be attributed to the aforementioned low political salience of formal privatizations, as well as to the Agenda for Change that foundation trusts usually adhere to voluntarily and thus employees keep their pay, terms, and conditions. A partnership agreement was concluded (IP22: 8–65) that was only relevant for the job evaluation process (IP22: 9–53). Nevertheless, the partnership was considered very successful (IP22: 7–62) and regarded as a showcase by UNISON (IP22: 8–62).

In the case of formal privatization of the GSTT, the preconditions necessary for the successful use of a partnership strategy (Fichter and Greer 2004) were not fulfilled. The binding institutional framework that guaranteed strong union and worker involvement was missing. Moreover, UNISON did not take a proactive role, nor did it use complementary strategies or embed the partnership strategy in a broadly appealing social agenda.

3.3.2 Findings: Germany

3.3.2.1 Background

Ver.di at the Vivantes hospital took a different approach than UNISON at the GSTT. Vivantes was transformed into a GmbH in 2001. The main reason for the formal privatization was the historical situation of Berlin. During the division of Germany, West Germany paid 50 per cent of the Berlin budget; consequently, Berlin was oversupplied with hospital beds in comparison to other urban centers. Due to reunification, Berlin was the most "inefficient" federal state with respect to its hospitals and employed the most personnel in comparison to all other states (Schwierz 2010). Therefore, both the management and the trade unions were aware of excess capacities and the necessity for closing hospitals and cutting personnel (IP28: 2–54, 30: 2–52). Nevertheless, this was taken as an opportunity by the trade union.

The process of formal privatization in Vivantes was triggered by a report from a health economist, commissioned by the Berlin Senate and paid for by the statutory health insurance fund AOK. The reason for the commissioning of the report was the increasing unwillingness of West German states to subsidize the Eastern states. The report thus looked for restructuring and cost containment solutions, and recommended to break up the municipal hospitals and to privatize them (IP31: 3–52, 5–57). Furthermore, formal privatization was a possibility for the state of Berlin to rid itself from infrastructure investment obligations that it had ceased meeting (IP24: 2–1810).

3.3.2.2 Resources and capabilities

Ver.di responded to the formal privatization in a proactive way, based on its strong institutional, but also associational power, by suggesting alternatives and threatening to appeal against the transfer of workers to the private company. Furthermore, it extended its strategic capabilities by commissioning an employee-oriented consultancy experienced with restructuring processes in the health sector.

For ver.di at Vivantes, the associational power resource of membership was not their main resource strength. However, it was a precondition for their confrontational strategy of appealing against the transfer to the corporation and their participation in the restructuring process, as will be outlined below. Trade union density in the Berlin municipal hospitals at the time of their formal privatization was at about "10 to 12, maybe 15 per cent".[2] This was perceived by a works councilor as a sufficient associational power basis to build up pressure (IP28: 18–47). In turn, the associational power resource of organization as a collective actor seemed to have been of greater importance. Within the hospitals, the trade union managed to establish a good communication structure and integrated the East Berlin works councilors by establishing a company-wide works council (IP28: 3–60, 4–66, 6–51). However, the fragmented structure of representation – each of the nine hospitals had their own works council – was a challenge. Some of the works councils of single hospitals resisted the transfer to the unitarian works council in the course of the merger into Vivantes because they did not want to give up their spheres of influence (IP28: 6–51, 6–58).

In accordance with the strong works council structures, institutional power resources, in terms of access to management, were generally good as well. Parts of the management had their own plans for the formal privatization. The administrative directors of the hospitals suggested forming a rather weak holding to avoid a restriction of their authority. This was opposed by the trade union as not sustainable (IP28: 4–59). The relation with the *majority* of the management was, however, cooperative from the beginning in the view of the works councilor, as they were willing to conclude an agreement guaranteeing no redundancies right at the start, regardless of the necessity to cut about 3,500 to 4,000 jobs (IP28: 13–66).

Ver.di in Vivantes had successfully pushed for commissioning the consultancy that specializes in works council consulting and moderation of restructuring processes in the hospital sector, thus enhancing its institutional power. The work of the consultancy was financed by the federal state of Berlin (IP28: 2). The relevant decision-makers agreed that all actors should be involved in a comprehensive merger and a formal privatization process of all of Berlin's municipal hospitals (IP31: 4–57). In this way, the heads of management included the works councilors, the ver.di shop stewards (Vertrauensleute), and ver.di activists of the different hospitals in a restructuring and corporatization process led by a consultancy (IP31: 4 Healthcare (57).

The resource of societal power was less important for ver.di. The management of the municipal hospitals cooperated with the Chamber of Industry and Commerce (Industrie- und Handelskammer, IHK) in the corporatization process (IP31: 4–61), but there was no cooperation between trade unions and civil society initiatives or other actors. According to a works councilor, this was unusual at that time (IP28: 12–61). Furthermore, access to the media did not play a major role. From time to time, the works council passed information to the media to increase the pressure (IP28: 16–60). Ver.di had good access to the Social Democrats since some of their activists in the sector were also members of the Social Democratic Party, who came into power in the state government during the corporatization process in 2001 (IP28: 12–60), and could presumably also exert some influence through this channel.

In terms of capabilities, ver.di framed the conflict in a pragmatic way and accepted the necessity to restructure the hospital landscape in Berlin (IP31: 6–66).

> Berlin [...] was the worst performing state with respect to economic efficiency and amount of personnel. It was clear from the beginning that

hospitals will have to be closed and personnel will have to be reduced in large quantities.

(IP28: 2–54)

However, ver.di did not restrict itself to a one-dimensional, market-oriented union identity. Its orientation to both market and society allowed the union to be more flexible in its strategies and extend its influence by credibly threatening to resort to militancy (IP28: 3–63). Furthermore, ver.di expanded its capabilities by commissioning the consultancy. Commissioning the consultancy entailed extended access to salient knowledge about the technicalities of restructuring processes, and it also introduced a deliberative element by the inclusion of employees into the process of restructuring (IP28: 2–57).

3.3.2.3 Strategies

The trade union's aim was to prevent the break-up and the privatization of the municipal hospitals (IP31: 3–52). This was done using a partnership approach, recognizing the restructuring process as an opportunity structure, suggesting an alternative concept, and bargaining over potential negative effects of the restructuring. The alternative concept suggested by ver.di included the merger of the Berlin municipal hospitals to strengthen them and avoid competition. In this way, they were to be enabled to be independent from subsidies and be profitable (IP31: 3–52, 3–58, IP28: 3–50). Furthermore, ver.di pursued the conclusion of a transfer agreement guaranteeing no redundancies.

The partnership approach was a promising option for ver.di at that time since the main interlocutor on the management side, the human resources manager, pursued a partnership approach as well and advocated communication, as well as exchange of arguments instead of confrontation (IP31: 10–58). Furthermore, the ver.di works councilor evaluated the cooperative approach to be the most influential:

> I would always try to reach an agreement. Because when it becomes a power game, you will achieve less since the employer side always has a greater leverage. It is just like that, even if the employees' side is well organized. That is why you always have to try and somehow find a compromise.

(IP28: 16–40)

The works council further promoted partnership work and increased its influence by including the aforementioned consultancy. The trade unionists were trained in the differences between the legal forms and the corresponding differences in codetermination rights and economic efficiency questions. This provided the basis for the trade unionists to become profoundly involved in the process and to bring in their expertise. Furthermore, the consultancy moderated the process, in securing the inclusion of both, employers and employees (IP28: 2–57, 8–51). The aim was to find a solution that was acceptable to all involved parties (IP28: 3–54). The cooperation of the works council and management went so far that they attended joint trainings led by the consultancy and went on study visits together to learn from other formally privatized hospitals (IP28: 8–65, 12–57).

Part of the restructuring process suggested by the union was a restructuring agreement (Überleitungstarifvertrag). The employer did not communicate openly that the restructuring process necessitated cuts in personnel costs by about 25 per cent, the equivalent of about 4,000 jobs. The trade union anticipated this and, thus, demanded the restructuring agreement. The trade unionists signaled that they were willing to accept job cuts since they acknowledged that capacities in their hospitals were above average and the hospital was therefore not profitable (IP31: 6–66). The adaptation of the hospitals, meaning a reduction in beds and a relatively higher reduction in personnel, was accompanied by work intensification (IP31: 7–64). The trade unionists nevertheless achieved a favorable agreement, with a guarantee for dynamic pay and pensions from the public hospital sector collective agreement, and no redundancies despite reductions in personnel (IP31: 9–66).

Ver.di also credibly threatened that it could resort to militancy if necessary. One of the most important means, and the only confrontational element that increased the union's leverage in the partnership and effects bargaining, was the use of the legal appeal against the transfer to the private company. Ver.di Vivantes collected all appeals and informed the employer of the number to put pressure on them and used it as a means to influence the Senate of Berlin members in negotiations. With the threat of appealing against the transfers to the GmbH, ver.di could negotiate favorable individual transfer contracts for their members (IP28: 12–63, 17–59, IP28: 3–63).

The ver.di trade unionists included their members from the beginning, also because the consultancy stipulated it. Works councilors of all hospitals, shop stewards, and ver.di activists of the hospitals were included (IP31: 4–55). Employees participated in project groups working on different parts of the restructuring process (IP28: 13–61). They also managed to motivate their members to follow their advice and appeal against the transfer of responsibilities, which bore some risk (IP28: 3–63). As mentioned above, these appeals helped achieve better transfer agreements (Überleitungsvertrag) for the employees (IP28: 15–47). They also paved the path for negotiations with the employer. Without this pressure, the trade unionists would not have been in the position to work with the management in partnership, but would have been forced to pursue a more aggressive strategy (IP28: 17–50). The Vivantes activists in single hospitals also oversaw the whole restructuring process with smaller activities, and the works council also organized meetings with employees (IP28: 13–54).

Last but not least, ver.di representatives also mentioned that cooperation with the parties, especially the Social Democrats, was important. They used their access provided by ver.di members that were Social Democratic Party members, too, to achieve additional leverage (IP28: 12–60). In relation to other strategies used, it nonetheless seemed to play a minor role.

3.3.2.4 Outcome

The whole transformation of Vivantes was perceived as a "success story" by the works councilor, both at the time and today (IP28: 6–54). The Vivantes trade unionists achieved their demand for security. They were willing to provide the necessary flexibility in exchange. There were no redundancies and no downgrading pay to lower bands; terms and conditions remained the same (IP31: 5–61). The newly founded GmbH joined the employer's association, and thus the validity of the public sector collective agreement was secured. Furthermore, the state of Berlin remained the sole owner of the hospital. Employees obtained extensive codetermination rights that granted them equal representation on the supervisory board. Moreover, working groups were established that would work on the hospitals' economic sustainability (IK 04/2001:33). Ver.di succeeded in building up enough pressure to achieve favorable transfers for employees by using the means of credibly threatening that large numbers of them could appeal against their transfers (IP28: 3–60). The necessary 3,500 job cuts out of 17,000 jobs in total were achieved in a socially responsible way, mostly through non-replacement of employees who retired. However, this could potentially have led to work intensification. Nevertheless, 98 employees of 13,500 remaining employees actually realized their threat and appealed against the transfer, meaning they were probably not satisfied with the transfer agreements ver.di negotiated with the employer (IP28: 2–65, 3–53).

Ver.di achieved the merger of all hospitals into one company to avoid competition between the hospitals. However, they had to accept the private legal form replacing the public legal form of an "Eigenbetrieb", one hospital was closed and two clinics were sold to the private company Helios (IP28: 3–60, IK 03/2014:47). Today, the former works councilor regards the demand to keep the legal form of an "Eigenbetrieb" as unnecessary if comparable codetermination rights are secured. "A GmbH in 100 per cent ownership of the state [...] is better than an 'Eigenbetrieb' in which [works councils] have weaker co-determination rights because you cannot participate in economic decision-making" (IP28: 9–50). Hospitals in private legal forms are economically more autonomous from the city council and state government, and this also increases the unions' scope of influence (IP28: 3–54).

There were no parts of the hospitals that were outsourced during the process, and the works council successfully claimed the right to codetermine about future outsourcing processes and negotiated that subsidiary companies of Vivantes needed to remain in at least 50 per cent Vivantes ownership (IP28: 6–54). Even though the merger and formal privatization process were regarded as cooperative and successful by the trade unionists, they noted that, in the aftermath, the establishment of a subsidiary and outsourcing of ancillary services, beginning in 2004 with the cleaning services, was a negative effect of the merger and formal privatization (IP28: 14–59).

Furthermore, it was regarded as a success that trade unionists and employees participated in the restructuring process (IP28: 6–54). However, due to the close cooperation, it was difficult for the works council to make their achievements clear, as the works councilor noted:

> [...] we missed one thing [...], we never understood how to sell our success. It was all invisible to the employees and the whole process was so rapid [...] I would not even have known how to sell them what we were doing in this committee.
>
> (IP28: 8–65)

Consequently, some works councilors were not re-elected into the new GmbH works council. "That was a clear sign that employees took some of our actions for evil because they did not grasp what would have been the alternative because it was difficult to convey" (IP28: 9–63). It might be concluded that ver.di was too influence-oriented and focused too much on partnership work, while not sufficiently including their members.

3.4 Comparison and conclusion

Contrary to traditional industrial relations theories, despite most-different institutional settings, trade unions in both cases studied pursued a partnership approach. This can be explained by common pressures stemming from marketization, as well as local-level organizational factors. The partnership approach matched the low politicization of the issue and its consequent pragmatic framing. Neither union regarded formal privatization as a highly contested issue, nor did they strongly oppose it, because of moderate effects for the workforce that they contained through agreements. However, ver.di at Vivantes acted more proactively and assertively, due to its greater institutional and associational power, and greater capabilities. It extended its capabilities, especially through the commissioning of the employee-oriented consultancy, in terms of information about the restructuring process, as well as deliberation with and inclusion of workers in the process. This also ensured their participation as a serious partner, which was additionally secured in a restructuring agreement. Furthermore, their trade union identity was oriented both toward market and society, and thus allowed the use of complementary, more confrontational strategies such as the legal appeal against the transfer of employees to the private company. Even though ver.di's framing was pragmatic, it was proactive at the same time. The union realized the opportunity structure the restructuring process provided. It used this opportunity not only to propose the inclusion of the consultancy but also to successfully set in motion a merger of the Berlin hospitals to reduce competitive pressure between them, as well as ensure their sustainability and eventually jobs. Therefore, in comparison, ver.di was able to exert greater influence on the process of formal privatization than its English counterpart.

In turn, UNISON at GSTT failed to secure one of the preconditions for successful partnership, the formalization of institutional power (Fichter and Greer 2004) and its access to management. UNISON could thus only get involved if it was in the management's interest. Furthermore, UNISON was not flexible in its strategic choice, also due to its one-dimensional local union identity. Thereby, it did not fulfil a second precondition for successful partnership. It was restricted by its strong market-orientation and self-concept as "conduit of information". This role was possibly taken because of the low politicization of the transformation into a foundation trust, but maybe also because of traditionally weak local trade union structures (Foster and Scott 1998). The mediator role and market-orientation also impeded the use of UNISON's traditionally high associational power in terms of union density to pursue more militant strategies, as well as their potential societal power to build coalitions and mobilize the public, given the strong public support for the public provision of health services in England.

The two cases confirm that success of partnership strategies strongly depends on the fulfilment of the preconditions put forward by Fichter and Greer (2004). They not only show the importance of a formalization of partnership but also demonstrate the importance of strategic flexibility and the enhancement of assertiveness through a combination of cooperative and adversarial strategies.

Notes

1. The AfC is a national agreement on pay and grading introduced in 2004 that replaced eleven previous national agreements that specified job grades, different allowances, and working conditions for different staff groups. They were replaced with only nine national pay bands, a job evaluation scheme, and harmonized terms and conditions. This also opened up work organization for local consultation and negotiation. However, further reforms from the mid-2000s, at least theoretically, contain elements that could erode the coverage of the AfC (Galetto, Marginson, and Spieser 2014, 9).
2. In German public hospitals, ver.di membership density is estimated at 23 per cent overall (Glassner, Pernicka, and Dittmar 2015).

References

Böhm, Katharina, Achim Schmid, Ralf Götze, Claudia Landwehr, and Heinz Rothgang. 2013. Five Types of OECD Healthcare Systems: Empirical Results of a Deductive Classification. *Health Policy* no. 113 (3):258–269. do.: 10.1016/j.healthpol.2013.09.003.

Collins, Ben. 2015. *Foundation Trusts and NHS Trust Mergers 2010 to 2015*. London: The King's Fund.

Doellgast, Virginia, and Ian Greer. 2007. Vertical Disintegration and the Disorganization of German Industrial Relations. *British Journal of Industrial Relations* no. 45 (1):55–76.

Esping-Andersen, Gøsta. 1990. *The Three Worlds of Welfare Capitalism*. Cambridge: Polity Press.

Fichter, Michael, and Ian Greer. 2004. Analysing Social Partnership: A Tool of Union Revitalization? In *Varieties of Unionism: Strategies for Union Revitalization in a Globalizing Economy*, edited by Carola Frege and John Kelly, 71–92. New York, NY: Oxford University Press.

Foster, Deborah, and Peter Scott. 1998. Conceptualising Union Responses to Contracting Out Municipal Services, 1979–97. *Industrial Relations Journal* no. 29 (2):137–150.

Galetto, Manuela, Paul Marginson, and Catherine Spieser. 2014. Collective Bargaining and Reforms to Hospital Healthcare Provision: A Comparison of the UK, Italy and France. *European Journal of Industrial Relations* no. 20 (2):131–147.

Givan, Rebecca K., and Stephen Bach. 2007. Workforce Responses to the Creeping Privatization of the UK National Health Service. *International Labor and Working-Class History* no. 71 (01):133–153.

Glassner, Vera, Susanne Pernicka, and Nele Dittmar. 2015. *Arbeitsbeziehungen im Krankenhaussektor, Project Report*. Linz: University of Linz.

Guy's and St. Thomas' NHS Foundation Trust. 2016. Annual Report and Accounts 2015-16. www.guysandstthomas.nhs.uk%2Fresources%2Fpublications%2Fannual-reports%2F2015-16-annual-report.pdf.

Halbwachs, Maurice. 1985. *Das Gedächtnis und seine sozialen Bedingungen*. Berlin: Suhrkamp.

Hall, Peter A., and David Soskice. 2001. An Introduction to Varieties of Capitalism. In *Varieties of Capitalism. The Institutional Foundations of Comparative Advantage*, edited by Peter A. Hall and David Soskice, 1–71. New York, NY: Oxford University Press.

Kahancová, Marta, and Imre Gergely Szabó. 2015. Hospital Bargaining in the Wake of Management Reforms: Hungary and Slovakia Compared. *European Journal of Industrial Relations* no. 2 (4):335–352.

Kaminska, Monika Ewa, and Marta Kahancová. 2017. State, Market and Collective Regulation in the Hospital Sector in East-Central Europe: Union Strategies against All Odds. *Comparative Labor Law & Policy Journal* no. 38 (2):257–289.

Keogh, Bruce. 2013. Review into the Quality of Care and Treatment Provided by 14 Hospital Trusts in England: Overview Report. London: NHS.

Kuehn, Bridget M. 2007. Global Shortage of Health Workers, Brain Drain Stress Developing Countries. *JAMA* no. 298 (16):1853–1855.

Kühn, Hagen, and Sebastian Klinke. 2006. Krankenhaus im Wandel. *WZB-Mitteilungen* no. 113 (2006):6–9.

Leys, Colin, and Stewart Player. 2011. *The Plot against the NHS*. Pontypool: Merlin Press.

Marrs, Kira. 2007. Ökonomisierung gelungen, Pflegekräfte wohlauf? *WSI-Mitteilungen* no. 09:502–507.

Obinger, Herbert, Carina Schmitt, and Stefan Traub. 2016. *The Political Economy of Privatization in Rich Democracies*. Oxford: Oxford University Press.

Schwartz, Hermann. 2001. Round Up the Usual Suspects!: Globalization, Domestic Politics, and Welfare State Change. In *The New Politics of the Welfare State*, edited by Paul Pierson, 17–44. Oxford: Oxford University Press.

Schwierz, Christoph. 2010. Expansion in Markets with Decreasing Demand-for-Profits in the German Hospital Industry. *Health Economics* no. 20:675–687.

Statistisches Bundesamt. 2016. *Grunddaten Krankenhäuser, Fachserie 12 Reihe 6.1.1*. Wiesbaden: Statistisches Bundesamt.

UNISON. 1995–2004. UnisonFocus. London: UNISON.

UNISON. 2004–2015. InFocus: The Monthly Magazine for All Activists. London: Unison.

ver.di Infodienst Krankenhäuser. 2001–2016. ver.di Niedersachsen-Bremen. http://gesundheit-soziales.verdi.de/service/publikationen/++co++b07f35e6-1f65-11e2-b271-52540059119e.

Vivantes. 2017. Portrait. http://www.vivantes.de/unternehmen/portrait/.

4 Negotiating outsourcing effects
Combining partnership and organizing strategies

4.1 Introduction

Outsourcing, contracting out, or functional privatization of support services in the health sector has a long tradition; however, the challenges for trade unions remain strong. Support services outsourcing is one of the earliest and most common forms of marketization in the hospital sector in Germany and England and it is well researched. The main reason for outsourcing support services in the hospital sector is cost containment realized through a reduction in personnel costs (Pollock 2004; Schweizer and Bernhard 2009). This is why contracting out of support services usually results in downward pressure on terms and conditions, job losses, and work intensification (Givan and Bach 2007, 139). The wages of the lowest-paid and most vulnerable (Walness 2002), and usually also female hospital staff, are eroded, reinforcing their peripheral status (Cousins 1988).

Furthermore, the threat of outsourcing undermines labor power (Pulignano, Doerflinger, and De Franceschi 2016), and outsourcing weakens union influence among hospital support services staff (Givan and Bach 2007, 140). It is challenging for trade unions to retain their outsourced membership (Foster and Scott 1998), and collective bargaining becomes more fragmented (see e.g. Doellgast and Greer 2007). In addition, unions are no longer benefiting from the state as a model employer, but are confronted with more hostile private employers (among others Givan and Bach 2007, 142). Last but not least, also care quality is negatively affected by outsourcing of support services (Davies 2005; Lethbridge 2012).

Due to these effects, trade unions have good reasons to try and prevent outsourcing, or at least to get involved in the process, assuring good collective agreements for their members, retaining their membership, organizing new workers, limiting the fragmentation of collective bargaining or, ultimately, insourcing the services. The challenges trade unions are facing not only in preventing outsourcing but also during the process and after are manifold and will be fleshed out in the following.

4.1.1 Challenges of outsourcing for unions

One of the main problems for trade unions with regard to the prevention of outsourcing is that outsourcing does not require consultation with worker representatives, and thus worker representatives have few formal tools to shape this reorganization (Doellgast and Greer 2007, 71). In Germany, unions were not able to prevent outsourcing in the hospital sector since the mid-2000s – in contrast to the 1990s – because of intensified cost pressures on wages (Glassner, Pernicka, and Dittmar 2015, 21).

Another challenge specific to the UK are the local trade union structures. An early study of municipal services outsourcing under the Conservative government between 1979 and 1997 in Britain by Foster and Scott (1998) emphasized that trade unions that only focused on national-level bargaining revealed their weakness when it came to local-level outsourcing. In turn, local trade union action can be used as an opportunity for union renewal if the trade union shifts its focus from servicing members to increased membership participation. When services are devolved or contracted out, and the local level is weak, trade unions are particularly vulnerable. In Britain, the national level of a trade union is usually in charge of campaigning while the local level is confined to peripheral matters of interpretation and is largely inactive (Foster and Scott 1998, 139).

Even if the trade union has sufficiently strong local structures, the organization and mobilization of workers before, during, or after the outsourcing process remains difficult. Outsourcing is a complicated and technical issue, especially in Britain (Foster and Scott 1998, 146), and of low political salience. According to Pollock (2004, 22 f.), it is a "less politically damaging way of cutting staff wages and of reducing terms and conditions than trying to dismantle national terms and conditions of service that had been agreed with unions". Especially when reforms are not justified ideologically by the government, but rather as a pragmatic end to the search for flexibility and low costs (as shown in the German telecommunications and automobile manufacturing industries (Doellgast and Greer 2007)), unions also tend to formulate a pragmatic critique, which might be less a mobilizing than an ideological critique (Givan and Bach 2007). Finally, ancillary workers have low public visibility, and thus receive little local attention in the press or in public debate (Cousins 1988, 221). Therefore, it is difficult to mobilize workers and the public to protest outsourcing in the first place. Another reason specific to the NHS might be a desensitization effect after competitive tendering in this sector has been practised for more than 30 years (also see Chapter 1).

Once outsourcing has been completed, unions are confronted with even greater challenges concerning the mobilization and organization of an increasingly diverse private and public sector workforce, as well as collective bargaining in the private sector.

First, being used to the state as a model employer, unions must tackle the challenge that employees might regard both their employer and themselves as victims of external pressures that forced the employer to outsource. A precondition for the activation of employees is that they attribute intensified workloads, job insecurity, and deteriorated terms and conditions to the discretion of the employer (Cunningham and James 2010).

Second, after the outsourcing has taken place, one of the biggest challenges Cunningham and James (2010) identified was that unions need to adapt their branch organization to accommodate workers in the privatized services. Usually, the outsourcing process leads to an increase in the number of workplaces, the organizational size becomes smaller and workplaces are geographically more dispersed. Unions have tackled this problem by establishing branches in some of the bigger organizations and by a workplace-related strategy that aimed to create self-sustaining membership groups at that level. Central to the success of this approach was that the union was perceived as having made a positive contribution to the employment protection of workers in the outsourcing process. The concern of workers about changes of terms and conditions in the aftermath of outsourcing has proven to be an opportunity for union membership growth (Cunningham and James 2010, 45 f.). However, it can also be a challenge. Marchington, Rubery, and Cooke (2004) and Doellgast and Greer (2007, 71) have shown that even in traditional union strongholds, not only in Germany but also in Britain, outsourcing has created pressure for concessions. Nevertheless, some unions successfully negotiated, for instance, release time for trade union activities in NHS contracting out (Givan and Bach 2007, 143).

Additionally, accommodation of workers in the privatized services is difficult since unions have a hard time keeping track of employees working for private contractors due to temporary contracts with short durations. The high turnover of staff also contributes to a difficulty in recruiting workplace activists, aggravated by intensive workloads, but also the aggressive manner of some managers (Foster and Scott 1998; Givan and Bach 2007, 146; Cunningham and James 2010). Moreover, as Cunningham and James (2010) found for the social care services, organization, and mobilization of workers in outsourced services is challenging since, on the one hand, there is a reluctance among transferred workers to take industrial action due to the public service ethos, and there is little understanding of the notion of collectivism among new workers in social care services who were not socialized in the public sector because of the low private sector unionization. Additionally, organizing workers in the privatized services is demanding since the original employer usually only grants facility time for union representatives to service members who are directly employed. In England, trade union stewards employed by the NHS are technically not supposed to represent contracted-out workers (Foster and Scott 1998). German works councillors do not automatically represent employees in subsidiaries either (§4 BetrVG). Furthermore, in Britain, unions might not be recognized by the private contractor (Cunningham and James 2010), and even despite union recognition, contractors in the NHS were also often unwilling to negotiate collective pay agreements (Givan and Bach 2007, 148).

Third, a problem specific to UNISON, traditionally the main English trade union in the public services, is its strong public service identity and lack of experience with organizing in the private sector.

Fourth, outsourcing also poses special challenges regarding collective bargaining. It leads to an increase in heterogeneity in workers' interests. First, outsourced workers are employed by another, private employer. Second, due to the transfer of undertakings agreements that only apply to transferred workers, new workers are subject to different collective agreements, pay, and pension schemes, as well as terms and conditions. The development of this so-called two- or multiple-tier workforce within the private companies is a major concern for trade unions. Even though competitive tendering began in 1983, it took until 2005, and the threat of the unions to withdraw their support from Labour, to reach an agreement to end the two-tier workforce in Britain (Givan and Bach 2007, 143, 146 f.). However, the two-tier code was withdrawn in 2010 (Cabinet Office 2010).

Foster and Scott (1998) identified and evaluated four trade union strategies, suitable to different extents in tackling the challenges associated with public service outsourcing that were elaborated in the previous section. The first strategy, industrial action, proved decreasingly effective against competitive tendering when the local trade union was not active enough. A second union response – although disputed within and between unions – was noninvolvement in the tendering process, following the rationale that unions should not actively engage in outsourcing processes to avoid legitimizing it, even partially. The third option of negotiating was a challenging one because of the above-mentioned weak local union structures and the complexity of outsourcing negotiations. When negotiating, Cousins (1988) also observed the dilemma between giving in to concessions to improve chances of in-house bids and the potential threat of losing jobs, as well as possibly even greater deterioration in terms and conditions if an external contractor wins. The success of cooperation with management depended strongly on the nature of management's approach and understanding with the unions, as well as on unions' organizational power (Cousins 1988, 221 f.). The only strategy that proved to be effective was legal remedies on the national level, the Transfer of Undertakings (Protection of Employment) Regulations (TUPE) that, in principle, secured transferred workers the same pay and conditions, and no less favorable re-employment. However, this regulation was amended and considerably weakened in 2014 (see Chapter 1 for more information).

This is why "beyond-the-workplace approaches", that were evaluated as a second promising strategy (Foster and Scott 1998), seem worth considering. In these approaches, unions relate to external constituencies, promote campaigns in alliances and increase pressure by making use of media. In her early study of competitive tendering in the NHS, Cousins (1988) identified a national-level strategy focusing on contractors' failures and reductions in service quality as a suitable issue for mobilizing the popular public support for the NHS. Cunningham and James (2010) recommended for the British social care services to combine workplace strategies, such as partnership with the employer and organizing workers, with beyond-the-workplace strategies that address external labor market and social concerns (Cunningham and James 2010, 37).

Departing from findings of the above-reviewed studies, some expectations can be formulated. First of all, given that the two cases studied in this chapter took place in two most-different settings, it could be assumed that trade unions choose differing strategies in the outsourcing processes. However, outsourcing poses the same challenges to unions at the local level that might outweigh the macro-institutional determinants. Since this form of marketization is moderately politicized and highly technical, and direct effects for members can be contained through collective bargaining, I expect that unions draw on their institutional and associational power to contain outsourcing effects instead of opposing it by deploying more adversarial strategies. Thus, they will pursue a combined partnership strategy, even though the inclusion of external constituencies by stressing beyond-the-workplace issues was evaluated as more adequate to contain outsourcing effects in the above-reviewed literature.

After having presented the challenges unions are facing, the strategies they have at hand during and after the outsourcing process, as well as my proposition for the cases to be studied, the findings of the two case studies will be presented. Finally, I will compare and discuss these findings.

4.2 Information on support service outsourcing cases

The comparison of the two recent cases of trade union strategies related to outsourcing processes in two large hospitals is embedded in a most-different systems design. Despite the comparable timing of outsourcing and strategies in the two cases, UNISON and ver.di were acting in the most-different national settings of healthcare systems and employment relations regimes. Regardless of these differences, both trade unions pursued a combined partnership and organizing strategy (also see Chapter 1 for more details on the overall research design).

The English case, concerning the Nottingham University Hospitals Trust (NUH), consists of two hospitals that employ 13,957 staff and have an annual turnover of £870m (2015–2016) (Nottingham University Hospitals NHS Trust 2016). Their cleaning services were outsourced in 2015. The NUH case was chosen because it is one of very few cases in which UNISON became involved in an outsourcing process, drawing on its newly established Strategic Organizing Unit (SOU) that is part of the national organization. UNISON called this case one of their biggest successes:

> The outsourcing of support services in the [...] Branch marks a special case in comparison with other outsourcings of support services in England since UNISON usually does not get active prior to the outsourcing and did not follow their membership into the private sector in the past.
>
> (IP20: 15–838)

Furthermore, this case was chosen because of its saliency compared to other cases of support services outsourcing, in which unions usually remained silent.

The German case took place in the biggest municipal hospital group in Germany, Vivantes. It arose from the merger of, today, 10 Berlin hospitals with about 5,471 beds, 14,714 staff, and an annual turnover of €1.02bn (2014) (also see Chapter 3). It also owns 13 care homes and two elderly residences, several outpatient facilities, as well as subsidiaries for catering, cleaning and laundry services (Vivantes 2017). The purchasing and logistics services, patient transport services, facility management, and therapeutic services of the Vivantes municipal hospitals in Berlin were outsourced in 2015–2016. The German case is a typical case since ver.di usually gets active when services are threatened to be contracted out and negotiates transfer agreements that secure terms and conditions. However, while in many municipal hospitals support services were outsourced earlier, Vivantes is a relatively late case of outsourcing (IP30: 18–308, IP24: 8–306).

The findings of this chapter are based on nine interviews (quotes from interviews marked as "IP") with full-time trade union representatives, but also local activists and works councilors, as well as the management. The analysis was complemented with a document analysis of the monthly publication "ver.di Infodienst Krankenhäuser" (IK) for the German case and the monthly publication "UNISON InFocus" magazine, the local UNISON NUH Facebook profile and newspapers for the English case (for more information on data generation and analysis see Chapter 1).

It should be acknowledged that the comparison is not straightforward since the English case deals with outsourcing of cleaning services only, while the German case also contains outsourcing of other services that include therapeutic services as well. However, all services in the German case were outsourced at once and can hardly be disentangled. Therefore, they are analyzed together. Nevertheless, the majority of outsourced services in Vivantes were ancillary services, and this case can still be regarded as a typical case that is in line with outsourcing and corresponding union strategies of other support services. In addition, local union structures in England are weaker than in Germany, and their own documentation of the rare struggles, as well as documentation in local newspapers, are scarce. This is the reason why an ideal comparison could not be found. Since outsourcing is of relatively low political salience and is barely reported in trade union or general media in England, and since trade unionists were less active and accessible than in Germany, this well-reported case was chosen for England.

4.3 Trade union responses to support service outsourcing

4.3.1 Findings: England

4.3.1.1 Background

The first important finding that helps understand and evaluate trade union strategies in the English support services outsourcing processes is that it is not as salient, and accordingly not regarded to be as important as other types of privatization by health sector unions. Judging from a document analysis of all issues of the "UNISON InFocus" magazine for activists from 2009 to 2014, all issues of the "Unite the Union: Workplace Reporter" from 2008 to 2014, as well as a complementary analysis of English local media, competitive tendering of support services was not a focus of trade unions in England. Between 2002 and 2015, 30 out of 348 articles (9 per cent) of the "UNISON InFocus" magazine related to marketization dealt with outsourcing in general, such as TUPE regulations, the two-tier code, or outsourcing-related Public Finance Initiatives (PFI), and only 10 articles (3 per cent) dealt with concrete cases that connected outsourcing with union activities, such as equal pay claims, prevention of outsourcing, or insourcing. This might be due to a habituation effect, because support services have been contracted out since the 1980s and campaigns in the beginning had limited success. Considering the strong protest against the Health and Social Care Act (HSCA) 2012, that introduced competitive tendering of clinical services, it can be assumed that it is also less salient because support services staff are not in direct contact with patients. Furthermore, in contrast to, for instance, the hospital sell-offs in Germany, contracting out of support services is reversible. Contracts are only commissioned for a limited period, and the hospitals can place a bid in the next round to bring the services back in house again. However, if a service is outsourced, the alternative public provider usually vanishes. Therefore, it is rare that services are brought back in house. Nevertheless, there are cases of insourcing when the private company cannot keep up with required quality standards (IP20: 7–712).

Since the NHS England has experienced numerous reforms and continuous marketization under all governments since 1979, trade unions had limited capacities and focused rather on scandalizing the use of PFI schemes or campaigning against the HSCA 2012 that enacted commissioning of clinical services. As a national UNISON trade union officer put it, "[…] our biggest thing was the campaign against the Health and Social Care Act [..] which we really saw as a big changing point" (IP06: 8).

Another reason why outsourcing on the local level was not accompanied by strong union campaigns might be due to the national-level trade union activities. On the national level, unions pushed for the introduction of the TUPE regulations and two-tier code that compensated the effects on workers, and therefore outsourcing was no longer a main concern of trade unions. However, these regulations were regarded as rather weak by the same unions and were even further diluted. Employers can circumvent regulations by re-evaluating jobs and downgrading their job description to a lower pay level or simply through intensifying work to reduce labor costs, or by not replacing workers who quit the job. New employees are recruited to a different pay scheme and are not covered by TUPE at all (IP21: 5–1466, 10–740, IP23: 9–1713, 11–13). As mentioned above, the two-tier code was withdrawn in 2010 (Cabinet Office 2010).

The private sector is an increasingly important field to organize in for UNISON. Nearly one-third of all new UNISON members are from the private, community, and voluntary sector, and membership in these sectors is growing most strongly (UNISON 2016, 5). Nevertheless, organizing outsourced workers and bargaining outsourcing effects are relatively new to UNISON. In the past, UNISON opposed outsourcing, but did not engage further once the outsourcing had taken place (IP21: 6–1464, 10–143). It was regarded as contradictory and tricky to first oppose outsourcing to private providers and later negotiate with the same provider that were first rejected (IP20: 10–1092). Today, however, UNISON calls itself the main union for NHS support staff (UNISON 2016, 33). At the national level, UNISON reinvigorated the One Team campaign that aims to raise awareness of the importance of support staff for the delivery of high quality patient care in the NHS (UNISON 2016, 32 f.). UNISON's aim across the four main private support service providers in the NHS (Capita, Carillion, Sodexo, and Steria) is to give workers a voice vis-à-vis the employer in a centrally coordinated forum (UNISON 2016, 7).

Additionally, UNISON observed a new wave of outsourcing since 2008 (IP21: 5–1466, 5–3282) that provoked increased efforts to organize outsourced workers. In the past, UNISON had not made a specific effort to follow its membership into the private services. This was due to a common view of the union that services should stay public. Only recently, UNISON "toned down [its] anti-privatization stance" (IP21: 14–78) and realized that it is not a successful strategy to "demonize" private employees, that they still deliver public services and should therefore be regarded as UNISON's responsibility (IP21: 14–78). UNISON had realized that it needed to get involved in outsourcing processes and to organize the privatized workforce as well. To this end, UNISON established the SOU at the national level. The SOU is the only unit in UNISON specifically working on behalf of outsourced workers (IP21: 1–3389). It comprises roughly 15 people (IP20: 1–512), and it gathers information on its membership in the private sector and the private providers (IP21: 2–122). The main aim is no longer to prevent outsourcing, but to preserve the membership. However, there is no automatism through which the SOU is informed about outsourcing initiatives. For this purpose, the unit resorts to monitoring, for instance, the Official Journal of the European Union and proactively approaches branches affected by public procurement of hospital services. However, only procurements that exceed a certain value are required to be published in the journal. Another possibility for the SOU to find out about the instances of contracting out is by being approached by their colleagues at the local level (IP20: 9–165). Carillion is one of four companies, together with Sodexo, Capita, and Prosteria, the SOU is focusing their work on, and with which UNISON has recognition agreements at the national level (IP21: 4–3128).

Regarding the concrete English case studied in this chapter, there were two main drivers for the Nottingham University Hospital NHS Trust to outsource its cleaning services. First, the trust's budget had a deficit (IP23: 2), and second, according to a trade union representative, services were not organized efficiently. Outsourcing cleaning services to Carillion gave the trust management the opportunity to pass the unpopular task of reorganizing the service and making it more efficient on to Carillion (IP23: 3, 15). UNISON first responded with a campaign, trying to fight off the contracting out. After the in-house bid had failed, the local branch received support from the national level, and UNISON shifted its focus from resistance to retaining membership and negotiating the transfer (STOP the Privatisation of NUH Services 2013a).

4.3.1.2 Resources and capabilities

UNISON at the NUH could draw little strength from membership density and public support, and benefited strongly from additional infrastructural resources provided by the national level.

Even though trade union density in the NHS is at a high level of an estimated 58 per cent (Pond 2006), the activation of this resource in the outsourcing process is difficult for unions. As a trade union officer stated, outsourced and transferred support service workers usually feel left alone by their union and quit. Members are also discouraged due to the long tradition of outsourcing of support services (IP21: 8–1821). After the outsourcing, it required additional support of UNISON's national-level structures to retain and recruit members, which turned out to be the strongest part of UNISON's associational power. The support came from two sources: the national-level SOU and the so-called "Fighting from Local" organizers (FFL) (IP23: 8–966). FFL organizers are trade union organizers who temporarily work in a branch to rebuild it (IP21: 2–3238). Usually, the national-level unit does not get involved in local-level campaigns (IP21: 9–2944), and their involvement is tricky due to a disconnect and prevailing mistrust between the different levels. The regional branches fear domination from the national-level unit and sometimes refuse to collaborate (IP21: 2–700, 3–1874). In contrast to other interventions by the national-level unit, FFL organizers are usually welcome in the regions and branches since they are an additional resource (IP21: 2–3238).

Based on national agreements, UNISON had a high level of institutional power. The union was accepted as the interlocutor by Carillion because it had a national recognition agreement with them, and it was more convenient than negotiating with the more militant trade union GMB, according to a UNISON trade unionist (IP23: 4f).[1]

UNISON also received some symbolic support in its anti-outsourcing campaign from its traditional ally, the Labour Party (STOP the Privatisation of NUH Services 2013a). However, UNISON's societal power resource was rather weak, even though UNISON tried to mobilize it by using online media and organizing various public events and protests in their anti-outsourcing campaign. In the post-outsourcing process, no societal power resources were used.

In the anti-outsourcing campaign, UNISON used a beyond-the-workplace framing, stressing that private companies had "no interest in the health of local people" (UNISON NUH Branch 2013). Such a campaign might have mobilized their societal power and brought about media coverage. How intensely and purposefully this framing was promoted and deployed to activate this resource cannot be evaluated in the realm of this study. However, it was obviously insufficient to prevent outsourcing of the services, perhaps because of weak local structures. Nonetheless, in the post-outsourcing campaign, UNISON focused on vested interests and organizing, and no longer aimed to mobilize the public.

UNISON showed a very market-oriented identity. The "gold-plated standard" of shop steward work as described by a member of the SOU included reporting the views of members to higher union levels – a "key contact of the democratic process" in the union, helping individual members with individual problems related to their work, and communicating problems to the local manager as a "spokesperson". Since the workload of a shop steward with this set of tasks is high, ideally, additional members are encouraged to become shop stewards (IP20: 12–2699). The definition of the ideal shop steward did not include adversarial or empowering elements, nor did it address beyond-the-workplace issues.

4.3.1.3 Strategies

Based on its resources and capabilities, the UNISON NUH Branch used different strategies to prevent outsourcing, but also to contain its effects. UNISON used political action and elements of social movement unionism in the outsourcing prevention campaign, and turned to an organizing and partnership approach afterwards. Strategies changed in the different phases of the outsourcing process and the analysis is structured accordingly.

In the beginning, in an effort to prevent the contracting out, the local and regional UNISON units mostly used political action and mobilization of the public. Their campaign "Stop the Privatisation" (IP23: 6–64) included comprehensive information on Facebook and the branch website, various events and protests, as well as a petition. UNISON received support of 1,298 signatories for a petition against outsourcing of the cleaning, catering, and porter services in 2013 (UNISON NUH Branch 2013); however, this number of signatories was too low for a successful petition. The activities were complemented by UNISON rallies (Howell 2013; STOP the Privatisation of NUH Services 2013b, c; Williams 2013) and public meetings with support of the Labour Party members who delivered speeches (STOP the Privatisation of NUH Services 2013a). Having a history of strikes against Carillion, members of the GMB union also voted for industrial action in 2013 (Bond 2013, Newman 2013). UNISON, however, refrained from industrial action. According to a trade union official, technically, UNISON could have organized a ballot among its members and gone on strike against outsourcing (IP21: 14–1368). This was, however, not considered in this case by UNISON. The reason remained unclear.

Even though UNISON framed their conflict at this stage as a beyond-the-workplace issue, they did not ally with other actors involved, nor did they succeed. The NUH Trust's in-house bid failed, and the protests and petition could not prevent the contracting out of the support services (Howell 2013).

Only after the local trade union campaign failed to stop the contracting out, the organization of workers started. UNISON's new national strategy was to organize workers in the biggest providers of the health sector, where a high density and recognition agreements already existed (IP 21: 4–3128). Part of this strategy was the provision of additional infrastructural support from the national level. The SOU retained members by talking to them, explaining their new contracts to employees, as well as recruiting and training trade union representatives in the outsourced service (IP21: 6–3166, 7–635, 8–1821, IP23: 9–1635). In addition,

UNISON demanded facility time (IP23: 1–796), and new staff was organized too (IP23: 8–0).

Unable to prevent the contracting out, UNISON turned to a partnership approach, focusing on securing terms and conditions based on the TUPE agreement with Carillion. The fear that the private provider would not negotiate with the union if it rejected outsourcing in the first place (IP20: 10–1092) did not realize in this case. UNISON was not branded as "anti-efficiency" (IP23: 4–495) as feared, and interviewees did not report difficulties in negotiating the transfer due to their former critical stance toward the private provider. Their switch in strategies did not pose a problem as such. However, in the transfer negotiations, UNISON was not recognized as an equal partner and Carillion remained the dominant party. Carillion agreed to keep the terms and conditions of the NHS as laid down in the TUPE agreement (IP23: 4–495), but found ways to circumvent them later (IP 23: 3–1889, 7–704).

4.3.1.4 Outcome

As a result of their strategic efforts, UNISON managed to retain their members and to organize some of the new workers. However, what followed were rivalries between old and new union representatives, deterioration of working conditions, and circumvention of TUPE regulations.

One of UNISON's main aims in the outsourcing process was to retain their membership. However, the SOU only became involved, and the most active trade union representatives were only recruited after the transfer had already been decided upon (IP21: 6–3166, 7–635). The local trade union representatives were then busy with servicing their members, for instance by doing case work and explaining new contracts to their members (IP23: 9–1635, IP21: 6–3166, 7–635). The UNISON NUH Branch also tried to organize the new staff that only joined Carillion after the transfer, but, as a trade union representative stated, they were only "slowly jumping on board" (IP23: 8–0), also because recruiters "could be more active" (IP23: 8–0). In the end, local trade unionists and the SOU managed to retain all existing members and gained 20 additional members. For the SOU unit, this was their "biggest success so far" (IP21:8–1821).

In terms of collective bargaining and representation structures, circumstances were naturally more favorable when the cleaning services were still part of the NHS. Carillion, like other private employers, negotiates collective agreements in a decentralized manner (IP34: 9–2944). Furthermore, it is difficult to represent outsourced workers since most union representatives are employed in the trust and not the outsourced companies (IP34: 4–1337). UNISON, however, achieved facility time for two Carillion trade union representatives for two days per week (IP23: 1–796). The trade union representatives are paid by the branches (IP23: 8–966).

However, even though these new representation structures at Carillion were an achievement for UNISON, they were also a challenge, since they created tensions between the original UNISON representative at NUH, who was

formerly responsible for the cleaning service, and the new Carillion representatives. NUH unionists tried to keep their activities as separate as possible from
the Carillion representatives (IP23: 9–0). Another problem was that the branch
secretary of the cleaning services was not TUPE-transferred and remained
employed by the NUH trust. However, Carillion wanted to deal with Carillion
representatives only and even provided them a union office on the Carillion
site, outside of the trust (IP23: 9–523, IP21: 7–2676).

With respect to the fragmentation of collective bargaining within Carillion,
there was differing perception of the existence and the extent of the problem
of workforce fragmentation in the so-called two-tier workforce. According to a
local Carillion trade union representative, this was not a major problem. New
employees were given the same terms and conditions, except that holiday and
sick pay only applied to them after six months. Thus, the divide in the workforce
was moderate. The underprivileged new employees were "just glad to have a
job" (IP23: 6–1312).[2] Two national trade union officials of the SOU, however,
reported that the creation of a two-tier workforce was one of the consequences
of outsourcing relevant to the union (IP20: 4–2219). In this way, it was difficult
in the 2014 NHS pay campaign to get all workers to sign a pledge about pay in
Carillion. The trade union's interest was to maintain advantageous terms and
conditions for the workers who were employed by the NHS, but, as a national
UNISON official put it,

> obviously, you've got people doing the exact same work and not being paid
> the same. And that's one of the biggest challenges in organizing the private
> sector, [...], you want to maintain the good things for your workers, but cre-
> ating two- or three-tier workforce[3] is like a nightmare to organize. How can
> you organize people that feel that they're unfairly treated?
>
> (IP21: 11–426)

After the outsourcing had taken place and transfers had been negotiated,
Carillion's willingness to cooperate turned out to have been merely a strategic
move, as previously assumed. After the transfer, UNISON representatives in
Carillion had the impression that the company was not open to their concerns
and that the employment relation had changed (IP23: 11). A Carillion trade
union representative for UNISON complained that Carillion management did
not openly communicate information (they're keeping their cards very close to
their chest) and tended not to consider trade union positions that were brought
up in consultations after the outsourcing (IP23: 2–293, 11–277, 14–101).

Furthermore, Carillion also circumvented the TUPE regulations. Working
conditions deteriorated through various mechanisms, as a new trade union representative of Carillion pointed out. Carillion's strategy was to not replace workers who left the job, which led to work intensification. Furthermore, Carillion
re-evaluated jobs and downgraded them, cut the unsociable hours enhancement and holidays (IP 23: 3–1889, 7–704). Also, customs and practices, such as
the practice of providing cabs for employees to get to a remote workplace, were
abolished (IP23: 3–1246). Carillion was said to "not do their job properly" (IP23:

10–555) due to a lack of experience. Consequently, due to work intensification, low pay and mismanagement, the morale among outsourced workers dropped. Workers felt that they were blamed for and had to "bear the brunt" of the financial deficit. These working conditions led to a high fluctuation in Carillion's workforce, with the result that they were "running on a skeleton crew. People just leave now" (IP23: 9–1713, 11–13). Due to the negative post-outsourcing developments, there was a notion that effects of the outsourcing were not contained through the TUPE agreement, but had to be bargained continuously (IP23: 7–704).

Altogether, membership was retained in the outsourcing process and a TUPE agreement was negotiated. However, workers were dissatisfied with working conditions under the new contractor, Carillion found ways to circumvent the TUPE agreement, and it did not recognize workplace representatives as equal partners. Continuous complaints about poor quality of services, expressed by the "Keep our NHS Public" (KONP) campaign group, not UNISON, eventually led to an earlier termination of the NUH and Carillion in April 2017 (Tengely-Evans 2016; Cooper 2017).

4.3.2 Findings Germany

4.3.2.1 Background

Also in Germany, outsourcing does not seem to be a highly politicized issue for trade unions. The analysis of the "ver.di Infodienst Krankenhäuser" showed that between 2001 and 2015, out of 118 reported conflicts that dealt with marketization of the hospital sector, only 15 (13 per cent) concerned outsourcing as a major issue, and in another three cases (2 per cent) it was a secondary issue (i.e. the main conflict concerned other forms of marketization). Ver.di reacted mainly with the partnership strategy (five cases), or a partnership through which they extended their influence with minor protest actions (four cases). More confrontational approaches were used in four cases, legal action in one case, and there was acquiescence in another one.

To understand the case of the most recent incidence of outsourcing in Vivantes, its long history of outsourcing and concessionary bargaining should be considered. The Vivantes GmbH was formed as a merger of the Berlin municipal hospitals in 2001. In the aftermath of this process, the cleaning, catering, and laundry services were outsourced to a subsidiary, but were still fully owned by Vivantes (IP30: 1–113, 1–619). The merger and outsourcing, however, could not prevent Vivantes from facing severe financial problems in 2004. The danger of bankruptcy was discussed and led to a coalition of the trade union, works council, employees and the state of Berlin that resulted in the restructuring agreement (IP24: 1–2428). In this "emergency agreement", valid until the end of 2016, employees sacrificed wages to allow for necessary restructuring and waived public sector collective agreement (TVöD) pay. However, giving in to pressure from the trade union, Vivantes rejoined the TVöD again in 2014 after years of bargaining. The management argued that the restored validity of the TVöD brought with it an increase in personnel costs of 2 per cent that needed to be contained by outsourcing services (IK 09/2014: 28f., IP30: 1–1679).[4] Therefore, the management was planning to further outsource parts of the hospital services – services, in which employees who formerly sacrificed their wages to give the hospitals a chance to restructure and restore their financial sustainability worked. The works council could prevent an immediate outsourcing by referring to the restructuring agreement (IK 09/2014: 28f.). Nevertheless, shortly after, the Vivantes board decided to outsource its therapeutic services into a newly founded subsidiary and to outsource its purchasing service and logistics, patient transport services and facility management into the existing Vivantes Service GmbH (VSG) (IK 12/2014: 52, IK 03/2015: 37, IK 09/2015: 28f., IP30: 2–1426). The VSG consisted, until then, of sterilization and laundry services (ver.di 2016b). In the next sections, the conflict will be analysed in more detail and the outcome will be presented.

4.3.2.2 Resources and capabilities

Similar to the English case, the resources of ver.di at Vivantes differed before and after the outsourcing. Ver.di at Vivantes had relatively low associational power pre-outsourcing, since it had limited personnel resources, and parts of the works council did not agree with ver.di's strategy. The union could compensate for this with the mobilization of employees for protest action. Societal power resources remained largely unused due to a predominant workplace framing. The use of resources in the post-outsourcing process, however, changed. Ver.di increased their leverage by increased unity, achieved additional infrastructural resources by working with a consultancy and widening its framing.

One of the main weaknesses during the conflict was ver.di's low associational power with respect to its ability to organize as a unified collective actor in the anti-outsourcing campaign. Unlike in earlier times, ver.di and the works council disagreed about how to respond to the outsourcing plans. Most of the works councilors were ver.di members, but formed their positions independently from ver.di and supported another strategy than the union of appealing against the transfer as laid down in the German Civil Code (§ 613a Abs. 6 BGB). Ver.di doubted the prospects of this strategy and preferred to conclude a collective agreement that would guarantee pay, terms, and conditions. Since only the trade union can negotiate collective agreements, ver.di was in the position to decide and enforce its strategy. Subsequently, ver.di officials had to make an effort to convince members of their strategy (IP30: 2–1783, 3–538, 4–712, 6–1253, 14–2265, 15–257).

Similarly, also (paid) personnel resources were limited despite high commitment of the trade union official responsible for the Vivantes hospitals. Furthermore, the secretary obtained support of another trade unionist, who coordinated a national service companies project in ver.di. This position, however, was not extended in 2016 (IP30: 13–762).

The ver.di official tried to compensate the lack of personnel resources, the lack of unity within the works council and low trade union density by building a strong workplace activist group that could organize itself and work independently (IP30: 13–762). Only 10 per cent of all Vivantes employees were ver.di members at that time, even though the numbers were rising slightly (IP30: 13–2575). The trade union official, and a representative of the activist group, also reported that since their members were used to being covered by the TVöD and having regular – seemingly automatic – increases in their wages, they were not used to fighting. The activists regarded it as a challenge to "shake people up" (IP30: 19–274) and to tell them they might lose their privileges if they did not start being active. Nevertheless, for protests and related activities during the outsourcing, ver.di managed to mobilize on average 80 to 150 of the 700 affected employees (IP30: 16–1027).

There was potential societal power, in the form of public support from Berlin inhabitants, that became visible in the Charité strikes for mandatory staffing levels (also see Chapter 6). The works council was counting on this support for the suggested appeal against the transfer from Vivantes to the GmbH but could not, as described above, convince the ver.di officials. Thus, this resource remained unused before the outsourcing took place, but was of more importance in the post-outsourcing campaign.

The perception of ver.di's institutional power, i.e. access to management and political decision-makers, differed between the works councilor on the one hand, and ver.di activists and their official on the other. Ver.di activists and their official mistrusted management and political decision-makers. They were concerned that the new employer would dismiss all employees who had appealed against the transfer, as suggested by the works councilor: "You cannot rely on them, that they won't do it" (IP30: 7–103). Therefore, they preferred to take preventive action rather than to trust the employer (IP30: 7–631): "We all know how it is with promises in politics – it is a question when they will be implemented and if they will be implemented at all" (IP30: 7–1326). For the trade union official and some trade union activists, it was clear that the board of Vivantes took the decision to outsource without consulting them and that the employees were not the board's primary concern (IP30: 7–2056).

The outsourced workers' structural power, more specifically, their workplace bargaining power, was perceived as high by the trade unionists, and their role was framed in empowering terms. Instead of referring to, for instance, the marketplace bargaining power of support service workers, which is relatively low due to the little qualifications required for their jobs (IP30: 6–294), or low associational power due to a low trade union density, trade unionists chose an optimistic framing and stressed the workplace bargaining power. This, in turn, was perceived as high because of the workers' determination to strike, and it proved to have a strong impact on the whole nature of the outsourced hospital services (IP30: 8–2082, 9–913). As the ver.di official put it, with respect to the sterilization services that are part of the VSG:

They are the 'bottleneck'. When we close it, nothing works anymore in the hospitals. Because then the whole business the hospital makes money with can only be held up for two more days at most until they have no surgery equipment anymore (IP30: 11–938). Patient transport services were regarded in this way as well (IP30: 3–2676, 8–2082).

The conflict as such, however, was framed only as a workplace issue by some of the ver.di activists and the responsible ver.di official. Their strategic orientation was therefore different from that of the works councilors. A ver.di activist stated: "Of course it is our aim to prevent outsourcing […] but we also have to take care of our members" (IP30: 8–3) who felt insecure about preventing outsourcing and wanted a transfer agreement that would secure their status. "Our ver.di position is […] clear: We want to prevent the outsourcing, would not mind reversing it, but in that moment, it was important that the people were secured" (IP30: 8–575). The ver.di official further argued that at the moment of the transfer, without a collective agreement, employees would have been affected by § 613a BGB, which means that they would have kept their TVöD conditions for only one more year. Their main aim was to achieve a certain degree of pacification and protection (IP30: 8–575). The works councilor was defeated with his alternative beyond-the-workplace framing that it was unethical for the federal states not to invest in hospital infrastructure because they are obliged to do so – which was, in his view, the real reason for the limited financial resources and the ensuing outsourcing plans (IP24: 2–1139).

After the outsourcing had taken place, ver.di increased its associational power again by jointly running a new campaign with the works council (IP30: 12–2258). The post-outsourcing Stand Together campaign aimed to increase personnel and implement staffing levels, to validate the TVöD in the subsidiaries and to insource the latter. Both ver.di and the works council felt obliged to stand united again (IP30: 17–2424). Ver.di also received additional funding for employing an external trade union consultancy that specializes in organizing and campaigning. Nevertheless, these resources were still judged as insufficient (IP30: 14–685).

The support of members was also crucial in the post-outsourcing campaign. The driver of the Stand Together campaign was the workers of the outsourced therapeutic services, who contributed considerably to creating the campaign (IP24: 5–446). A trade unionist explained this with their professional self-concept: They regard themselves as part of the medical services, responsible for the patients, and thus being outsourced like cleaning services was perceived as inappropriate (IP24: 8). However, they were solidary with support service workers.

Furthermore, this time the potential societal power was also used. The Stand Together campaign was timed to exert maximum political pressure during the 2016 state elections in Berlin (IP24: 5–2452, 7–1208). Furthermore, the union officials and representatives of Vivantes cooperated closely with their colleagues at the Charité and joined forces in the joint campaign Uprising of Subsidiaries (Aufstand der Töchter) (ver.di 2017c) which happened after the end of data collection.

4.3.2.3 Strategies

Ver.di's strategies can clearly be divided into a pre- and a post-outsourcing phase. To prevent outsourcing, ver.di focused on protests at board meetings, while it combined effects bargaining with increased confrontation in the post-outsourcing phase. The union also started to cooperate with the Charité activists who struggled with similar problems and explicitly targeted the public with their actions.

Before the outsourcing was decided upon, ver.di mainly focused on a number of smaller protests with employee participation (IK 09/2014: 28 f., IK 03/2015: 30, IK 06/2015: 37, IP30: 16–2023, 16–510, 17–438, IP24: 3–448, 3–3509). Vivantes also addressed an open letter to the Vivantes management and the Senator of Health Mario Czaja pleading against outsourcing (IP30: 16–2023, IP24: 3–1923). These actions could have been suitable to mobilize the public, but seemed to fail in doing so. The works council also engaged in lobbying, particularly of the Social Democratic Party (IP30: 7–695, 16–1842, IP24: 3–1526). The main target of union action at this time seemed to be the supervisory board meetings. After outsourcing had been decided and the implementation process was being planned, ver.di organized small protests, supported by on average 80 to 150 employees, for each meeting of board members throughout the entire year (IP 30: 16–510, IK 12/2014: 52). After every supervisory board meeting, ver.di published press releases (IP30: 17–438). However, all these activities were not able to prevent the outsourcing.[5]

When outsourcing was regarded as inevitable, ver.di started to engage in bargaining over effects and increased pressure by using more confrontational elements in 2016. The union also pushed effects containment further by demanding the insourcing of all subsidiaries in 2017. For this purpose, it started a joint campaign with activists from the Charité Facility Management (CFM), the support services subsidiary of the Charité hospital, who were struggling with similar issues and addressed the public more intensely.

Ver.di's first reaction after the outsourcing decision had been taken was effects bargaining by means of negotiating a transfer agreement (IK 06/2015: 37). Ver.di's demand was to keep all regulations from the public sector agreement, TVöD, for current workers and automatically adopt future amendments. Additionally, ver.di demanded no redundancies until the end of 2019. The municipal employers' association, did not support these demands in the beginning, but the bargaining partners soon came to an agreement after ver.di threatened to go on strike (IP30: 3–2676, 8–2082).

Shortly after the negotiations of the transfer agreement were concluded, the works council and ver.di engaged in extended effects bargaining. In 2014, only 70 per cent of all employees in Vivantes and its 14 subsidiaries were employed under the TVöD. Except for one subsidiary, there were no collective agreements. Also, working conditions were rated as deficient according to a survey conducted in the two cleaning subsidiaries (IK 09/2015: 28). The aim was to secure the same working conditions for all employees. To this end, ver.di started with a week of action at the end of November 2015 (IK 12/2015: 21–22, IP30: 11–242, 11–1374, IP24: 5–446, 5–2452). After the employer failed to make an acceptable offer for a collective agreement from the VSG, the union resorted to confrontation to extend its leverage and called its members out on a warning strike in June 2016. It was supported by a majority of 95 per cent of all members in the ballot, and, eventually, 400 of 700 workers of the VSG and many therapists directly employed with Vivantes went on strike. Initially, it was planned for two days, but lasted for 15 days in the end. Matching its framing and its recognition of the structural power in the process of production, ver.di focused on the sterilization services during their strike. Vivantes and the VSG, however, undermined the strike by sterilizing medical equipment in other hospitals. Nevertheless, since the externally sterilized equipment was not usable for reasons of low quality, Vivantes eventually had to cancel lucrative elective surgeries. Subsequently, in the second round of bargaining, the management was more cooperative (IK 06/2016: 24 f., IK 12/2016: 32) (rbb 2016).

To raise support for collective bargaining, ver.di communicated with its members at high levels in Vivantes and called for regular works meetings (Betriebsversammlungen) to inform members, but also to organize new workers of the Service GmbH (IP30: 5–658, 11–242, 11–1374, 12–449, IP24: 3–883, 6–172). The whole Stand Together campaign rested on organization and mobilization of members (IP30: 12–449), which was also reflected in the collaboration with the union consultancy (IP30: 12–1631). Especially the demand for more personnel and higher staffing levels in Vivantes necessitated an increase in union density and greater support from employees, since the demand could not be realized under the TVöD, but required an in-house agreement with Vivantes. Therefore, ver.di made its work conditional on increasing membership levels (bedingungsgebundene Tarifarbeit) (IP30: 19–1531). With this strategy, ver.di gained enough members in the Service GmbH to build a bargaining committee and start negotiating with the employer (IK 12/2015: 22). Organizing was also crucial to ver.di due to aforementioned limited personnel resources (IP30: 13–543, 13–2072) and a relatively low trade union density.

Ver.di at Vivantes increased its adversarial orientation by joining forces in the Uprising of Subsidiaries campaign with their colleagues from the Charité (ver. di 2017c). It was a reaction to the hospital employers, who collaborated as well (Supe 2017). The objective of this campaign was public sector pay for all workers and insourcing of all outsourced services at both Vivantes and the Charité. Part of the campaign involved joint warning strikes at the beginning of 2017 (ver.di 2017c). After collective bargaining at Vivantes failed, more than 90 per cent of affected members voted for an unlimited strike (Strandt 2016). The strikes led to an escalation of the conflict[6] but not to a breakthrough. Further confrontation followed (ver.di 2017d), however, it did not yield to success. The union maintained its demands, but shifted its focus on public sector collective bargaining, abolishment of the DRGs, introduction of needs-oriented staffing levels, and demands related to the Covid-19 pandemic (ver.di 2020).

4.3.2.4 Outcome

Ver.di obviously could not prevent the outsourcing of Vivantes' purchasing and logistics services, patient transport services and facility management into the existing VSG, as well as its therapeutic services into a newly founded subsidiary. However, the aim of the outsourcing was cost containment through lower personnel costs, but cost savings were limited for Vivantes (IP30: 5; IP24: 1f). Ver. di managed to contain effects on current employees' wages and conditions. The union achieved a collective agreement securing all current employees in the outsourced services a dynamic validity of the TVöD and excluding redundancies until the end of 2019 (IP30: 3–2676). Therapeutic service workers with permanent contracts remained employed directly by Vivantes (IP30: 17–1995, 1–2245). Thus, cost savings could only be obtained from new employees who were no longer paid according to the TVöD standard (IP30: 10–184). Furthermore, ver. di at Vivantes successfully mobilized its members for strike action and started close collaboration with their colleagues at CFM, increasing its associational and societal power.

However, the collective agreement was not supported by all members, because of the divide between works council and ver.di officials and activists. Especially in the outsourced patient transport services, members were upset (IP30: 3–2676, 8–575). Consequently, the works councilor argued that with the conclusion of the agreement, ver.di accepted both the establishment of the GmbH and the transfer of employees, thus opening the door to further outsourcing and corporatization in the form of GmbHs. Moreover, the works councilor criticized that new employees were not included in the agreement (IP24: 3–2385, 4–1736, 4–2695).

The ver.di official, activists and works council were later jointly striving for the TVöD to be valid for all workers in the subsidiaries in the Stand Together campaign. The campaign also aimed to bring about a general increase in personnel and staffing levels and insourcing of all subsidiaries (IK 09/2015: 28 f., IK 06/2016: 40; IK 09/2016: 24 f., IK 12/2016: 32). Ver.di started negotiating over a collective agreement for the approximately 1,000 Service GmbH employees and was successful at mobilizing a considerable number of workers for a strike (ver.di 2016a) (IK 12/2015: 22). Given the high mobilization potential of members in the warning strike, ver.di estimated that potentially about 500 beds would need to be closed during the strike (IK 06/2016: 24 f., IK 12/2016: 32) (rbb 2016). The Stand Together campaign was then turned into the joint Uprising of Subsidiaries campaign with the Charité, where workers of the CFM subsidiary were striving for public sector pay levels for all employees and insourcing of the subsidiary as well. Strikes were coordinated and thus publicity and pressure increased (IK 06/2016: 24 f., IK 12/2016: 32) (rbb 2016, ver.di 2017c).

In the course of these post-outsourcing campaigns, ver.di achieved the return of all workers who had been outsourced into the VSG in 2016. However, 268 of 900 employees working for the VSG are employed directly through the subsidiary and without a collective agreement (ver.di 2017b). After the end of data collection for this case study, negotiations for a collective agreement in the VSG could be achieved in 2018 after 51 days of strike. It guarantees 90 per cent of public sector pay and other public sector conditions (ver.di 2018). However, the union did not succeed in insourcing the subsidiary until 2020 and seems to have shifted its focus.

4.4 Comparison and conclusion

Comparing the two cases of outsourcing, it could be observed that both unions faced the usual challenges of outsourcing. There was no requirement to consult with worker representatives about outsourcing, and unions struggled with a relatively low salience of the issue. In both cases, unions used partnership and organizing, as well as elements of social movement unionism, but in differing orders. UNISON started out with a campaign that might have had developed toward social movement unionism, and retreated to partnership post-outsourcing. Ver.di acted the other way round. The union first concluded a transfer agreement, a partnership approach, and turned to more confrontational tactics post-outsourcing. With its strikes in the Uprising of Subsidiaries campaign, ver.di showed that support service workers can increase their low public visibility, and outsourcing can be an issue of public attention. The beyond-the-workplace strategy was suitable for mobilizing workers and gaining media leverage. The strategy was suitable for containing outsourcing effects at least in parts.

Both unions managed to deal with the challenge of increasing fragmentation by adapting their local union organization to accommodate workers in the privatized services. UNISON negotiated facility time with the new provider, and the union officers received their own office. However, the fact that the NHS was no longer responsible proved to be a challenge, and there were tensions between the old and new works councils. In the German case, the original ver.di works council still regarded itself as responsible for outsourced workers. UNISON also showed that it was able to adapt to its changing membership structure. While Foster and Scott (1998) still found that UNISON's public service identity impeded the union from taking action in outsourcing and representing outsourced workers, UNISON officers meanwhile acknowledged the growing importance of activity in the privatized services. This was also expressed in the establishment of the SOU and the fact that UNISON now calls itself the main union for the NHS support staff (UNISON 2016, 33).

UNISON's associational power resources were strong pre-outsourcing, given its high union density in the hospital services. Furthermore, the local union received additional support from the national level, and therefore could retain members and even organize some new recruits post-outsourcing. In its pre-outsourcing campaign, UNISON tried to draw some strength from its societal power resources, but was not successful. The union only received some symbolic support from the Labour Party, but did not manage to mobilize public support in the pre-outsourcing campaign despite a beyond-the-workplace framing. This might be due to weak local structures that have only been strengthened by the support of the national SOU in the post-outsourcing process. Another explanation for the failed activation of societal power resources might be UNISON's strong market-orientation that pays little attention to societal or class interests. UNISON's pre-outsourcing campaign might have had the potential of serving as a basis for social movement unionism, but the union failed to cooperate with other actors, despite Labour Party support. UNISON abandoned this approach after the outsourcing had taken place and also refrained from other confrontational measures such as industrial action.

In contrast to UNISON, ver.di's associational power was relatively weak pre-outsourcing, because of a division over strategic choices between works council and trade union officials. The union's other associational and infrastructural resources were only limited, and it tried to compensate for this by strengthening the activist core in the workplace.

Eventually, UNISON did not prevent outsourcing, but, on the whole, retained membership and secured terms and conditions. These achievements, however, needed to be permanently fought for. Carillion circumvented TUPE regulations by re-evaluating jobs, and working conditions deteriorated. A two-tier workforce of transferred and newly recruited workers emerged, which had negative effects on the 2014 pay campaign. Furthermore, UNISON developed a more self-confident understanding of its role. The union gave up its stance that it was not possible to first oppose outsourcing and then bargain about its effects with the new provider. The union negotiated with Carillion and implemented representation structures. However, the representatives reported that they were not taken seriously by the Carillion management, and information was not communicated to them. This might be attributable to a lack of formalization. UNISON failed to use its high density and did not try to mobilize members. Its organizing and partnership strategy was not qualified to sustainably and permanently secure working conditions, pay and representation structures. This might be again due to a lack of formalization of the partnership and due to organizing that only focused on recruitment, but failed to mobilize members for collective action. Furthermore, a complementary strategy, containing more confrontational action in order to be recognized as an equal partner, was lacking. UNISON also never took into consideration reversing outsourcing. Lastly, in contrast to what Foster and Scott (1998) found for the municipal services, the reliance on legal remedies was not the most effective strategy for UNISON in the studied case since the TUPE agreement had been diluted, and the two-tier code had been withdrawn.

In contrast to UNISON, ver.di intensified confrontation in the post-outsourcing process. The union increased its associational power by aligning strategies with the works council and drawing on additional support of the union consultancy. Furthermore, Vivantes support services workers joined forces with their colleagues from the CFM, and started drawing on the potential societal power present in the state of Berlin. The union started using beyond-the-workplace framing and pursued a social movement unionism-oriented strategy. When ver.di went on a joint strike with the CFM, structural power also came into effect. In comparison to the English case, ver.di engaged in more extensive effects bargaining and showed a stronger belief in agency than their English counterpart.

In both cases, outsourcing could not be prevented or be reversed by the unions. However, ver.di seems to have been more successful in mediating negative effects for workers of the outsourced services. Furthermore, ver.di increased its power resources post-outsourcing and managed to mobilize members for strike action and the public for a campaign. This could only be achieved because the union did not shy away from adversarial strategies, practicing membership inclusion from the beginning, as well as a beyond-the-workplace framing.

Notes

1. There is low competition between the trade unions since only UNISON has a recognition agreement with Carillion (IP21:11–2796). UNISON collaborated with the GMB and Unite in the TUPE transfer (IP23:11–1720).
2. The fear for unemployment cannot be explained with an unusually high unemployment rate in the region. In 2016–2017, 4.7 per cent of the working population in England were unemployed, while only 4.1 per cent were unemployed in the East Midlands (Office for National Statistics 2017).
3. When using the term three-tier workforce, the SOU refers to the following three forms of employment in outsourced services: (1) Workers transferred under the TUPE framework, who retained the terms and conditions under the AfC due to negotiations by the union. They are employed on NHS contracts but managed by the private contractor. (2) Workers who are directly employed by the contractors. (3) Agency staff deployed by the private contractors (IP20: 16–1286).
4. The trade unionists rather held the federal state of Berlin and its lack of investment in hospital infrastructure responsible for Vivantes' financial deficits (IP24: 2–1810), which the Vivantes management also admitted later (IK 09/2016: 24 f.).
5. As mentioned above, the works council pursued an alternative but outnumbered strategy of appealing against the transfer of workers to the subsidiaries at that time. The logic of the strategy advocated by the works council was that if all 700 employees that were about to be outsourced appealed against their transfer, this would be highly politicized and the state of Berlin would not risk the negative publicity, or the public would put pressure on the city council. The idea was that this could eventually prevent the outsourcing of the services. The works council was aware of the risk that employees who appealed could lose their job if the state of Berlin did not give in to the potential public pressure (IP24: 3–2385, 4–1736, 4–2695). In this case, employees would have been covered by the TVöD terms and conditions for only one more year (Nachwirkung) (IP30: 7–575). Furthermore, the works council wanted to file a complaint against the state of Berlin because it did not fulfil its obligation for infrastructure investments – for him, the actual cause of the cost pressure (IP24: 2–2987).
6. The Vivantes management canceled the negotiations and banned ver.di and all workers on strike from entering the facilities in one of its hospitals (ver.di 2017b). Furthermore, Vivantes made a successful case in the labor court that ruled the warning strike was an unlawful political strike since it demanded insourcing – a decision protected by entrepreneurial freedom. Ver.di could ward off consequences by arguing in front of the court that this demand was directed at policymakers and not management (ver.di 2017a).

References

Bond, Katie. 2013. Union Members Vote for Action. *Swindon Advertiser*, October 31.
Cabinet Office. 2010. Two-Tier Code Withdrawn. https://www.gov.uk/government/news/two-tier-code-withdrawn.
Cooper, Ben. 2017. Hygiene Standards at Nottingham's Hospitals Increase from the Lowest to Highest Rating. *Nottingham Post*, December 15.

Cousins, Christine. 1988. The Restructuring of Welfare Work: The Introduction of General Management and the Contracting Out of Ancillary Services in the NHS. *Work, Employment & Society* no. 2:210–228.

Cunningham, Ian, and Philip James. 2010. Strategies for Union Renewal in the Context of Public Sector Outsourcing. *Economic and Industrial Democracy* no. 31 (34).

Davies, Steve. 2005. *Hospital Contract Cleaning and Infection Control.* London: UNISON.

Doellgast, Virginia, and Ian Greer. 2007. Vertical Disintegration and the Disorganization of German Industrial Relations. *British Journal of Industrial Relations* no. 45 (1):55–76.

Foster, Deborah, and Peter Scott. 1998. Conceptualising Union Responses to Contracting Out Municipal Services, 1979–97. *Industrial Relations Journal* no. 29 (2):137–150.

Givan, Rebecca K., and Stephen Bach. 2007. Workforce Responses to the Creeping Privatization of the UK National Health Service. *International Labor and Working-Class History* no. 71 (01):133–153.

Glassner, Vera, Susanne Pernicka, and Nele Dittmar. 2015. *Arbeitsbeziehungen im Krankenhaussektor, Project Report.* Linz: University of Linz.

Howell, Dominic. 2013. Demonstrations to be Held Over QMC and City Hospital Privatisation Plans. *Nottingham Post*, October 25.

Lethbridge, Jane. 2012. *Empty Promises: The Impact of Outsourcing on the Delivery of NHS Services, Technical Report.* London: UNISON.

Marchington, Mick, Jill Rubery, and Fang Lee Cocke. 2004. Prospects for Worker Voice across Organizational Boundaries. In *Fragmenting Work: Blurring Organizational Boundaries and Disordering Hierarchies*, edited by Mick Marchington, Damian Grimshaw, Jill Rubery and Hugh Willmott. New York, NY: Oxford University Press.

Newman, Andy. 2013. First Anniversary of GMB Strike Action against Carillion. *Socialist Unity – Politics. Culture. Debate.* https://socialistunity.com/first-anniversary-of-gmb-strike-action-against-carillion/?utm_source=rss&utm_medium=rss&utm_campaign=first-anniversary-of-gmb-strike-action-against-carillion.

Nottingham University Hospitals NHS Trust. 2016. Annual Report & Accounts. https://www.nuh.nhs.uk/media/2327108/0230_nuh_annual_report_2015-16_web.pdf.

Office for National Statistics. 2017. A01: Summary of Labour Market Statistics. https://www.ons.gov.uk/employmentandlabourmarket/peopleinwork/employmentandemployeetypes/datasets/summaryoflabourmarketstatistics.

Pollock, Allyson. 2004. *NHS plc: The Privatisation of Our Healthcare.* London: Verso.

Pond, Richard. 2006. Liberalisation, Privatisation and Regulation in the UK Healthcare Sector/Hospitals. http://www.pique.at/reports/pubs/PIQUE_CountryReports_Health_UK_November2006.pdf.

Pulignano, Valeria, Nadja Doerflinger, and Fabio De Franceschi. 2016. Flexibility and Security within European Labor Markets: The Role of Local Bargaining and the "Trade-Offs" within Multinationals' Subsidiaries in Belgium, Britain, and Germany. *ILR Review* no. 69 (3):605–630.

rbb. 2016. 900 Mitarbeiter von Charité und Vivantes im Streik http://www.rbb-online.de/wirtschaft/beitrag/2016/04/Charite-vivantes-berlin-warnstreik-aufruf.html.

Schweizer, Lars, and Barbara Bernhard. 2009. Strategische Optionen öffentlicher Krankenhäuser Zwischen Markt und Hierarchie – Eine Empirische Studie. In *Vernetzung im Gesundheitswesen: Wettbewerb und Kooperation*, edited by Volker E. Amelung, Jörg Sydow and Arnold Windeler. Stuttgart: Kohlhammer.

STOP the Privatisation of NUH Services. 2013a. Public Rally against Privatisation. October 24 [Facebook post].

STOP the Privatisation of NUH Services. 2013b. Public Rally against the Privatisation of Nottingham University Hospitals Services [Facebook event].

STOP the Privatisation of NUH Services. 2013c. SECOND Public Rally against the Privatisation of Nottingham University Hospitals NHS Services [Facebook event].

Strandt, Steffen. 2016. Aufstand der Töchter hat begonnen. https://www.sozialismus. info/2016/08/aufstand-der-toechter-hat-begonnen/.

Supe, Johannes. 2017. Wieder gemeinsam gestreikt: Arbeiter zweier Klinikservicegesellschaften protestierten vor Charité-Hauptsitz. Junge Welt. https://www.jungewelt.de/artikel/ 307524.wieder-gemeinsam-gestreikt.html.

Tengely-Evans, Tomáš. 2016. NHS Victory in Nottingham Hits Privateers Carillion. *Socialist Worker, November 29.*

UNISON. 2016. UNISON Annual Report 2015/16. UNISON. https://www.unison.org. uk/content/uploads/2016/04/23784.pdf.

UNISON NUH Branch. 2013. StopThePrivatisation [Petition]. https://www.change.org/ p/stoptheprivatisation.

ver.di. 2016a. Stand Tarifverhandlungen Vivantes Service GmbH. http://gesundheit-soziales-bb.verdi.de/branchen-berufe/krankenhaeuser/vivantes/++co++7bbcecfc-c869-11e6-8abe-525400940f89.

ver.di. 2016b. Vivantes Service GmbH. *Pressemitteilung.* https://bb.verdi.de/presse/ pressemitteilungen/++co++eff6485e-2ca9-11e6-8ed5-525400a933ef.

ver.di. 2017a. Hintergründe zum Streikverbot. https://gesundheit-soziales-bb.verdi. de/branchen-berufe/krankenhaeuser/vivantes/++co++9682a414-113e-11e7-848f-525400940f89.

ver.di. 2017b. Streikverbot für Vivantes Service GmbH. https://gesundheit-soziales-bb.verdi.de/branchen-berufe/krankenhaeuser/vivantes/++co++8549be12-0fef-11e7-92ed-525400ed87ba.

ver.di. 2017c. Warnstreik VSG und CFM. https://gesundheit-soziales-bb.verdi.de/ branchen-berufe/krankenhaeuser/vivantes/++co++19f02e6e-0bd8-11e7-8c8a-525400ed87ba.

ver.di. 2017d. Was passiert in der VSG? https://gesundheit-soziales-bb.verdi.de/branchen-berufe/krankenhaeuser/vivantes/++co++c9b7cce0-279d-11e7-9b65-525400ed87ba.

ver.di. 2018. Streik endet nach 51 Tagen: Tarifergebnis für Vivantes Service Gesellschaft. https://www.verdi.de/themen/nachrichten/++co++7520ff2a-64d3-11e8-9e19-525400940f89.

ver.di. 2020. Krankenhäuser in Berlin verschaffen sich Respekt: Erfolgreiche Warnstreiks bei Charité und Vivantes. https://gesundheit-soziales-bb.verdi.de/++file++ 5f7dba6242cd9528eb59c949/download/201001_Flugblatt%20Charit%C3%A9%20 mit%20Layout.pdf.

Vivantes. 2017. Portrait. http://www.vivantes.de/unternehmen/portrait/.

Walness, Derek. 2002. *Securing Our Future Health: Taking a Long-Term View.* London: HM Treasury.

Williams, Dylan. 2013. 'Don't Sell Us Out To The Lowest Bidder': Job Fears At QMC and City Hospitals. *Impact - The University of Nottingham's Official Student Magazine, October 27.*

5 Resisting medical service privatization*
Exploiting market specificities and high salience

5.1 Introduction

Material privatization usually marks the end of a longer process of marketization that involved, among others, corporatization and outsourcing. It is defined as a change in ownership from the public to the private sector. In comparison to corporatization, that concerns the legal form of a hospital, and to outsourcing, that usually concerns support services, privatization involves the transfer of the core task – the medical treatment – to a private provider. Although there were no privatizations of whole hospitals in England, medical services were subject to functional privatization, i.e., the contracting out or outsourcing of a medical service to a for-profit service provider. Due to the common character of these two privatizations and the common core of transferring the core task to the private sector, they will be treated as functional equivalents in this chapter.

Studies from Britain (Foster and Scott 1998), Canada (Jalette and Hebdon 2012), and Germany (Greer, Schulten, and Böhlke 2013) show that unions can respond to privatization using any number of tactics: public campaigning through: (1) mobilizing members in demonstrations, strikes, and other actions; (2) mobilizing allies in politics and civil society; (3) using legal levers, such as litigation or arbitration; or (4) influencing change in conversation with decision-makers through proposing alternatives and/or detailed participation as comanagers. These options are available in both Germany and England. Jalette and Hebdon (2012) find in a survey of Canadian municipalities that the selection of these tactics matters: proposing alternatives and using several tactics simultaneously were more likely than industrial action to prevent privatization from taking place. However, as Glassner, Pernicka, and Dittmar (2015) have argued, health system-specific differences affect industrial relations. As will be shown, the two countries differ in terms of two different constraints facing privatizers, which serve as levers for campaigners.

* This chapter is largely based on joint research with Geneviève Coderre-Lapalme, University of Birmingham, Department of Management, g.coderre-lapalme@bham.ac.uk, and Ian Greer, Cornell University, School of Industrial and Labor Relations, icg2@cornell.edu.

The main political constraint for NHS privatization is that it can be framed as a threat to a national health system; in Germany's decentralized mixed economy of hospitals that includes public, private for-profit, and private not-for-profit providers (see Chapter 1), this is more difficult. In both countries, most large-scale privatization initiatives are of high salience, attract noisy protests, and public scrutiny, which generate uncertainty and unwanted publicity for firms and policymakers. In Germany, in turn, there is a separate, highly technical discussion of funding and regulation that anti-privatization campaigners have had little success influencing.

In addition, there are health system-specific organizational constraints and, consequently, potential political opportunity structures. Purchasing bodies in the NHS are relatively new and inexperienced, have unclear roles under the statute that created them, and are subject to a complicated regulatory system that subjects commissioning to a series of approvals from other parts of the NHS (IP40, IP41). The elected leaders of German municipalities and states, by contrast, have clearly defined and well-established roles set out in a written constitution. Furthermore, when a contract in England comes to an end, the service can easily be won in the next iteration by an NHS provider, and contracts can also be terminated by either side; the transfer of a German hospital into private ownership, by contrast, is intended to be permanent. NHS purchasers are therefore more susceptible to the tactics of campaigners than German state and local politicians, and NHS privatization decisions are more reversible.

Power resources, such as access to decision-makers, institutional leverage, high membership density, and supportive civil society are important resources for unions. Health unions generally possess strong power resources. As Table 5.1 shows, the populations of both Britain and Germany overwhelmingly support government provision of healthcare, and this support has held steady over time. In 2006, 4.5 per cent of West Germans told the International Social Survey Programme that the state should "definitely not" or "probably not" "provide

Table 5.1 Perceived government's responsibility to provide healthcare

Year	Country	Definitely or probably should	Definitely or probably should not
1985	West Germany	97.6%	2.4%
	Great Britain	99.1%	0.9%
1990	West Germany	95.4%	4.5%
	East Germany	98.9%	1.1%
	Great Britain	99.2%	0.9%
1996	West Germany	96.6%	3.4%
	East Germany	99.1%	0.9%
	Great Britain	98.5%	1.5%
2006	West Germany	95.5%	4.5%
	East Germany	97.3%	2.7%
	Great Britain	98.9%	1.2%

Source: ISSP, "do you think it should be or should not be the government's responsibility to provide healthcare for the sick?", various years.

healthcare for the sick". In East Germany, this figure was 2.7 per cent and in Britain 1.2 per cent. Support for public provision of healthcare is, thus, a little higher in Britain than in Germany, and support for the NHS might be even stronger due to its creation as part of national solidarity after the Second World War which is still present in the "collective mind" (Halbwachs 1985; Baggott 2004, 86 ff.). As is shown below, in both countries, there is potential of citizens willing to protest the privatization of health services.

Based on the above, in both countries, campaigns can be expected to benefit from strong public support and high associational power. They have an incentive to draw on this societal power and to frame their campaigns in terms of a social agenda beyond their members' self-interest. English campaigns may, on the one hand, benefit from a particularly high political salience of medical services outsourcing due to its novelty and historic origin of the health system, as well as due to inexperienced purchasing bodies and, in addition, from high trade union density. On the other hand, English health sector unions may suffer from a fragmented union landscape. German unions may, in turn, benefit from unity and strong local structures. However, they are characterized by lower trade union density and will face strong and experienced political actors. They will have difficulties in politicizing the change in ownership from public to private since private provision has always been a pillar of healthcare in Germany.

After having assessed the challenges unions are facing in the course of medical service privatization and the outlook of possible anti-privatization strategies, the cases studied in this chapter will be presented, compared, and discussed.

5.2 Information on medical service privatization cases

The chapter compares several major privatization initiatives of medical services respectively whole hospitals in two most different settings of healthcare and employment relations institutions. Cases in this chapter are defined as trade union strategies designed to combat privatizations of medical services respectively whole hospitals. Success is defined as the prevention of such initiatives (also see Chapter 1 for more details on the overall research design). All privatizations followed a particular change to the law aimed at increasing competition between providers: the introduction of the diagnosis-related groups (DRGs) reimbursement system in 2003 in Germany and the introduction of competitive tendering of medical services by Clinical Commissioning Groups (CCGs) through the Health and Social Care Act (HSCA) in 2012. The timescale was chosen because these two changes were both frequently named by interviewees as unleashing a wave of health service privatization initiatives and campaigns against them. All large-scale privatizations of hospitals in Germany with more than 900 beds since the introduction of the DRGs were examined, as well as all medical service outsourcings with a value above £60m. Smaller NHS commissioning exercises or hospital privatizations in Germany with fewer than 900 beds were left out, as well as privatization initiatives that did not lead to anti-privatization campaigns. The cases include campaigns involving unions either as leaders or followers. Success or failure is defined in terms of whether or not privatization took place and not in terms of outcomes such as wages, working conditions, union power, internal union management, collective bargaining coverage, or health spending.

The German cases are constructed from interviews with trade unionists, managers, elected officials, and consultants carried out in 2003–2004, 2006–2007, and 2015–2016, as well as ver.di's periodical "Infodienst Krankenhäuser" (IK) and media sources. The first round included 27 interviews, mostly in Hamburg (to date, the largest example of hospital privatization in Germany), but also at the national level. The second round included sixteen interviews examining hospitals elsewhere, some of which had been restructured without being privatized. The third round included seven interviews focused on more recent campaigns in Dresden and Schleswig-Holstein.

The English case studies are based on interviews with the same mixture of respondents, carried out in the wake of the 2012 HSCA, in 2012–2013 and 2014–2015. The first round of 30 interviews was focused on the effects of the Act on private sector firms and NHS purchasing practice, but because of the noisy politics of the reform also included information on unions and other campaigners. The second round of 15 interviews concerned trade union campaigning.

5.3 Trade union responses to privatization and commissioning of medical services

5.3.1 Findings: England

In England, national unions fought marketization and privatization together, starting with their opposition to the Health and Social Care Bill of 2011. The British Medical Association, the Royal College of Nursing and the largest Trades Union Congress (TUC)-affiliated healthcare trade unions, Unite and UNISON, joined with the main health journals, including the British Medical Journal, the NHS Confederation, several health policy academics, "non-aligned" health policy think tanks such as the King's Fund and Nuffield Trust, as well as the House of Commons Health Select Committee, which was led by a Conservative former health secretary, to express concern with the bill (The Times 2011). The TUC's All Together for the NHS and UNISON's 999 campaign began as efforts to coordinate lobbying and then spilled over into future efforts to safeguard the NHS (TUC 2011). Campaign groups 38 Degrees and Save Our NHS organized online petitions, asked members of the public to lobby their member of parliament to vote against the Bill, organized events around the country and declared 1 April 2011 "All Together for the NHS" day (Hood 2011). Unions also tried to get different interest groups to sign open letters to the government, including the royal colleges and health charities, but this proved difficult, and some withdrew following pressure or promises from the Department of Health (IP40).

After the Bill received royal assent in March 2012, NHS restructuring remained highly politicized. Demonstrations were organized, both locally and nationally, in collaboration with campaign groups, unions, Labour Party activists,

Table 5.2 Anti-privatization campaigns in England

	Name	Value[1]	Year	Outcome
1	Bristol CCG mental health services	210m	2014	Privatization avoided
2	Weston-super-Mare	–	2014	Privatization avoided
6	George Eliot Hospital	–	2014	Privatization avoided
3	West Sussex musculoskeletal services	235m	2014	Privatization avoided
4	Dorset pathology	60m	2014	Privatization avoided
5	Cambridgeshire Adult Care	800m	2014	Privatization avoided
6	Staffordshire cancer services	1.2bn	2015	Privatization avoided

1 Source: UK government contracts finder archive https://data.gov.uk/data/contracts-finder-archive/. Figures were not available for Weston or George Eliot.

and members of the public. UNISON's 999 campaign organized demonstrations to oppose cuts in the NHS and threats of privatization and supported strikes by NHS staff (UNISON 2013). Trade unions also supported the August 2014 People's March for the NHS, in which thousands of NHS staff, trade unionists, campaigners, and activists marched 300 miles from Jarrow to London, to raise awareness and to oppose NHS reforms and cuts (Jenkins 2014). In the 2015 general election, Labour made defending the NHS from privatization its principal issue (Robinson 2014).

Spurred on by concrete threats of local privatization by the new CCGs and the example of Hinchingbrooke, numerous local anti-privatization campaigns took place. Many were led by local trade unionists, some with expert advice, legal support and information from their national union (IP40, IP42). Others – this could not be observed in Germany – were led by grassroots groups, in some cases supported by groups such as 38 Degrees, which helped coordinate volunteers and meetings and in providing information. These tended to be successful. In this section, all cases of large-scale medical services outsourcing with a value above £60m from 2014 to 2016 will be presented (see Table 5.2).

In Bristol, campaigns with limited trade union involvement took place where the CCG was looking to tender out mental health services. The main campaign group, "Protect our NHS" (PoN), was involved very early in the process, having been setup immediately after the creation of the Bristol CCG in late 2012. Those who joined were mostly local activists, keen to stop private sector involvement in the delivery of local NHS services. When the CCG decided to commission services for the first time in 2013, PoN became regulars at public CCG meetings, to question the decision-makers and put pressure on them in order to keep services in public hands. In parallel, they organized actions in coalition with trade unions and other community groups, with the main argument that private sector profits had no place in the NHS, while both questioning the quality of their current services and noting their aggressive tax planning arrangements (PoN 2014). Tactics included petitions, picketing, and handing out leaflets, but also more creative actions: a flash mob choir at Bristol Hospital, a rock concert, giant posters, and a crowd-funded documentary (IP42, IP43). The campaign gained momentum with local media, with the BBC reporting on public CCG meetings (IP43) (Hill 2014). However, trade unions in Bristol remained relatively quiet in their support compared to PoN activists, and there was little participation other than being present at some public events (IP43, IP44, IP46). This is in part due to work intensification for staff and branch representatives, which made them less likely to mobilize, the risk of harming relations with employers and unspoken pressures in keeping a low profile (IP46). Campaigning was led by PoN with some cooperation with the unions' local health and regional branches.

Despite substantial public support, PoN activists found themselves progressively shut out of CCG decision-making. They decided to take legal action in early 2014 over the CCG's procurement policy, which they considered unlawful, as it should have made provisions for public consultation (Hill 2014). The CCG was forced to change its policy after a judicial review and, during the same period, published a shortlist of tenders for mental health services, which excluded all private providers that had been interested in the contract.

In Weston-super-Mare, PoN was also involved in campaigning following the decision by the North Somerset CCG in 2013 to contract out the management of Weston General Hospital. The context in Weston-super-Mare was different than in Bristol, however, with the population being more conservative and difficult to mobilize. Nonetheless, different groups worked together to stop the private takeover and restructuring of the hospital. This included PoN, the UNISON local government branch, the Patients before Profits campaign group, "Keep our NHS Public" (KONP) and some professionals from the local health branch (IP43, IP45). Although mobilization was more difficult, the coalition still managed to be heard in a process which again intended to shut out public consultation. Successes in Bristol also gave some strength and momentum to Weston-super-Mare campaigners. The CCG eventually decided in mid-2014 to only consider public sector bidders, despite notable private sector interest (UNISON 2014b), and the local Conservative parliamentarian expressed support for this decision (Wright 2014).

Trade unions led some of the other successful campaigns. At George Eliot Hospital in Nuneaton, the same model as Weston and Hinchingbrooke was proposed as a solution to underperformance in 2011, promoted by the Trust Development Authority (TDA) tasked with guiding restructuring (BBC 2013). When in 2012 it became apparent that the TDA would push for contracting out to the private sector, Unite decided to lead a campaign called "Hands off GEH" (IP42). The national union sent staff experienced in leading successful campaigns to work with local activists to setup stalls at the local market, hand out leaflets and initiate picketing and petitions. Campaign leaders were active in speaking to the media to pressure the TDA to keep the hospital in public hands. There was also some collaboration with other groups, although collaboration between the campaigns led by UNISON and Unite remained loose (IP42). The Labour Party and its local candidate ran their own campaign called "Keep GEH part of the NHS" to use this local issue to win votes in the upcoming general election (Malyon 2015; Swinford 2015).

Unite campaigners received strong support from the national union, and, unlike non-union campaigners, they did not have to rely on crowd-funding or scrape together donations (IP42). They deployed a "beyond-the-workplace" framing and argued that the private sector would put profits before patients, which would then lead to cuts in services available and distort the patient/doctor relationship (UNITE 2014). The campaign culminated with a group of Unite-backed activists picketing in front of the TDA offices in London on the day a decision was to be made on tenders. They were unexpectedly invited to a discussion with TDA decision-makers, and the purchasing process was canceled in March 2014. Although the TDA cited the hospital's improved financial performance, both UNISON and Unite trade unionists argued that in this case, without their own campaigns, the franchise would have gone ahead (IP42).

A series of successful local campaigns followed in 2013–2014. Beyond those mentioned already, campaigners managed to keep services out of private sector hands, for example, in West Sussex (musculoskeletal services), Dorset (pathology), Cambridgeshire (adult care) (Leng 2014; Stretton 2014; Ryan 2015). Campaigners in these cases used various tactics, mostly involving the mobilization of union members and proposing public sector alternatives to CCGs. Most included coalitions of diverse local activists, with union branches supporting local anti-privatization campaigns. Since then, several tendering projects have been put on hold (IP40).

The largest commissioning exercise in the English sample, a 10-year contract for cancer care services in Staffordshire, worth around £1.2bn, was on hold from 2014 due to a campaign (BBC 2014). Grassroots campaigners collected 70,000 signatures for a petition against the private sector takeover, which brought media attention and prompted local governments to raise their own concerns, leading councilors to vote against the proposed privatization (BBC 2015; Express & Star 2015). The CCGs' decision over providers was planned for December 2015 but did not take place (UNISON 2016). Unions supported the "Cancer not for Profit campaign" and wrote to NHS Chief Executive Simon Stevens, demanding an end to the commissioning exercise (UNISON 2014a).[1] After the end of data collection, the contracting out of the Staffordshire cancer services was eventually given green light in the end of 2016 by NHS England (BBC 2016). However, the CCG Governing Bodies decided not to proceed with the contract award. On their website, the commissioners explain:

> Through extensive engagement with patients and carers commissioners have learned that there is excellent clinical care in Staffordshire and Stoke-on-Trent, but services are not joined up and there is insufficient co-ordination between professionals and the different providers of care.
>
> (NHS 2017)

Instead, the CCGs decided to improve coordination between professionals and the different providers of care in Staffordshire and Stoke-on-Trent.

In the case of NHS community services across Bath and North East Somerset, Virgin Care won a contract of more than £700m in November 2016. Eventually, the Conservatives holding a majority within the Bath council voted for the deal to go ahead. Both commissioning exercises took place after the end of data collection.

All six campaigns analyzed led to the collapse of the commissioning exercise. Campaigners argued that it was unethical for private sector providers to make profits from the ill health of the British population and would often use the example of the US healthcare models as a way of illustrating the potential costs of NHS privatization. They applied tactics such as legal challenges, picketing, and influencing decision-making by attending CCG meetings. Unlike Germany, it was not always trade unions who took the lead. This is due to limits to union action (for instance, overwork of local branch activists, fragmentation of national unions and lack of a strong local union structures), as well as due to the longstanding politicization of health policy and a wave of campaigning that brought numerous members of the public into activist roles following the 2012 Act.

Campaigners had more tools at their disposal than their German counterparts. They could, for example, seize on flaws in the process due to the lack of experience of CCGs, as in PoN's campaign in Bristol. In other cases, such as in West Sussex, private providers withdrew because of commercial concerns. Many campaigns were successful because of strong grassroots organizations and good cooperation of these organizations, and because of the unions originating from a stronger salience of the topic in England. Political factors were most important: George Elliot and Weston General were politically sensitive large hospitals, whose restructuring would take place in the shadow of the 2015 general election. As polling firm Ipsos Mori reported on the eve of the election,

> one area where the government needs to tread very carefully is health services. Fear for the future of the NHS is at the highest level we've measured, and the risks are very real for the government if they are seen to damage one of the UK's most treasured institutions.
>
> (Mori 2015)

The exception is again Virgin Care winning a contract of more than £700m in November 2016 to run NHS community services across Bath and North East Somerset. Financially, this is so far the largest contract a private health company has ever won from a single authority (Cameron 2016). PoN campaigned to stop this initiative, but their protests and petitions failed, even though comparable to the successful campaigns in Bristol and Weston. The large contract won by Virgin Care in late 2016 may reflect a learning process on the part of purchasers or the government's increased confidence following its 2015 general election victory.

5.3.2 Findings: Germany

In Germany, unions became involved in health financing policy only after the most important changes had taken place. Ver.di, which had just been formed in 2001 through a merger of the public sector union "Gewerkschaft öffentliche Dienste, Transport und Verkehr" ÖTV with four other service sector unions, organized a campaign called "Gesundheitskampagne" in hope of influencing the 2002 bill that established DRGs. This campaign was an experiment, and lawmakers took the union's advice only "in homeopathic doses" (ver.di 2003). Based on lessons from that experience, later campaigns were more successful. Ver.di achieved an increase in hospital financing in 2008 with its campaign *Der Deckel muss weg* (IK 10/2008), and, through the *Der Druck muss raus* campaign, ver.di has brought the issue of understaffing (stemming from DRGs and insufficient government investment) to the attention of federal lawmakers (IP37). Furthermore, starting in the 1990s, ver.di and ÖTV were involved in several campaigns that aimed to counter privatization due to excess capacities after reunification, some also involving the Marburger Bund. In this section, all privatizations of hospitals with more than 900 beds since 2003 will be examined (see Table 5.3).

Most of the German campaigns against cases of large-scale privatization were unsuccessful. The largest case of privatization in Germany was Hamburg's public hospital chain, the "Landesbetrieb Krankenhäuser" (LBK). Asklepios Kliniken purchased a majority stake in 2004 despite strong worker and community mobilization. Ver.di and a wide range of allies from civil society organized a non-binding referendum, in which the overwhelming majority voted against privatization. The state coalition government of the Conservative Party and right-wing populist Schill Party overruled voters, citing financial concerns including LBK's debt. This was followed by an unsuccessful campaign of the

Table 5.3 Anti-privatization campaigns in Germany

	Name	No. of beds	Year	Outcome
1	Landesbetrieb Krankenhäuser-Hamburg	5,150	2004	75% sold to Asklepios
2	Universitätskliniken Marburg-Gießen	2,377	2006	95% sold to Rhön
3	Klinikum Krefeld	1,023	2007	Sold to Helios AG
4	Universitätskliniken Schleswig-Holstein	2,265	2003-2010	Privatization delayed
5	Regio Kliniken Kreis Pinneberg	938	2009	Sold to Sana
6	Städtische Krankenhäuser Dresden	1,529	2010	Privatization avoided

Source: Own presentation, number of beds from German Hospital Register (DKV) http://www.deutsches-krankenhaus-verzeichnis.de/ (2016).

same actors to render referenda in Hamburg legally binding. Demonstrations and work stoppages with the aim of linking working conditions and pay to the public sector collective agreement, TVöD, followed. The coalition here was extremely broad and had a wide range of social justice issues, such as the local provision of health services which is not guided by profit orientation, but also including a focus on local democracy. This was a deliberate choice by ver.di and the local DGB, as a response to their exclusion from policymaking under the new government (Greer 2008). Protests were fueled by the reputation of Asklepios as more of a hardheaded commercial organization than its main competitors (IP25). A collective agreement linked to the public sector framework was achieved in 2007 and codetermination organs at the corporate level were set up (IK 03/2002, 02/2003, 06/2003, 09/2003, 11/2003, 07/2004, 11/2004, 10/2005, 12/2005, 06/2006).

The university hospitals Marburg-Gießen were the second largest hospital privatization; a Conservative-led state government planned their privatization in response to heavy indebtedness. Trade unionists, supported by the civil society alliance "Rettet die Klinika", tried to fight off privatization, but participated in a planning group of the Conservative government at the same time. This campaign focused more on health system and workplace issues but also pointed to the risks of private provision that might lead to the abolishment of unprofitable units of the hospital, a decrease in the number of beds and longer waiting lists for surgeries (Wulff 2005). In 2006, the hospitals were sold to Rhön-Klinken AG (which the parent company of Helios purchased in 2013 for €3.03bn (Siebelt 2013)). Afterward, ver.di took industrial action – strengthening the union's own organization and its political connections – and achieved a collective agreement with Rhön (IK 07/2005, IK 03/2006, IK 06/2006, IK 04/2008).

In 2007, the municipal hospitals in Krefeld, North Rhine-Westphalia, were sold off to Helios by the municipal coalition government of the Conservatives and Liberals (Freie Demokratische Partei, FDP). Ver.di successfully collected enough signatures among the local citizens to initiate a referendum on the privatization of the Krefeld hospitals. Despite ver.di's preparations for the referendum, a lawsuit and suggestions for alternatives, the municipal hospitals were privatized (IK 06/2007, 12/2007) (RP Online 2007).

In a very similar way, the publicly owned Regio-Kliniken of Pinneberg in Schleswig-Holstein were sold off to Sana by the municipal Conservative-Liberal coalition government in 2009 due to accumulating deficits stemming from rapid expansion and specialization. The sell-off took place as the alliance "Pro Regio-Kliniken", consisting of ver.di, Social Democrats, Greens and the Left, was still collecting signatures for the initiation of a referendum. Politicians pushed privatization through quickly, before reliable figures on the economic status of the municipality or the auditor's report were made public (IK 10/2009) (Augener 2009; Kolarczyk 2009).

Ver.di did succeed in two cases. In the university hospitals of Schleswig-Holstein (UKSH), where privatization has been under consideration since 2006, the union staved off privatization, again not without concessions. This discussion was particularly sensitive since employees had been sacrificing their wages since 2005 for hospital restructuring. In the negotiations for another concessionary collective agreement, ver.di went on strike and included non-privatization in their demands. Subsequently, in 2008 ver.di won a clause that prevented privatization until 2015. In exchange, ancillary services were outsourced into a fully-owned subsidiary (Service Stern Nord GmbH), and the political decision about privatization was postponed to April 2015. The Conservative-led state government broke the latter agreement by preparing the privatization already in 2010, citing financial considerations. Ver.di protested this breach of the collective agreement, with the support of the Social Democrats and Greens, and argued that this threatened both the largest employer and the largest hospital. Instead of privatization, the government opted for a public-private partnership in 2010, based on the British model. Ver.di made alternative suggestions, supported – as in Minden – by the employee-oriented consultancy BAB Institut, but failed due to a lack of power and exhaustion from years of struggle (IP32, IP34; IK 06/2010, IK 12/2010). Nevertheless, privatization was not discussed again since then, possibly because the public-private partnership eased the financial pressure and the state government changed from Liberal-Conservative to a Social Democratic-led in 2012.

In Dresden, ver.di anticipated privatization, based on experiences in other cities, and worked to prevent it. The Conservative mayor and the Conservative majority in the municipal government attempted to convert the municipal hospitals into a publicly owned corporation (GmbH) as a response to poor financial performance and a need for investment. This was opposed by an alliance of Social Democrats, Greens, Left, ver.di, and works council. Ver.di argued that full privatization would threaten patient care since a private provider would be more profit-oriented, and it pointed to the recent privatization of the municipal housing company and its negative effects. After an overruled referendum on this matter, ver.di successfully lobbied for a new ordinance, making referendum outcomes legally binding for three years. The alliance initiated a referendum over both the GmbH form and privatization of the hospitals; voters rejected both. Since then, all parties have successfully engaged in restructuring the hospitals to avoid privatization (IP35, IP29; IP36; IK 03/2012).

Four out of six of the German campaigns did not prevent privatization (Table 5.3). In these cases – Hamburg, Marburg-Gießen, Krefeld, and Pinneberg – ver.di mobilized members and allies in a political campaign against privatization, but the campaigns were ignored by the Conservative politicians making the decisions. The other two campaigns were successful: in Schleswig-Holstein because of a strike and concessionary deal; and in Dresden because of an unusual preventative legal and political strategy. It was crucial for the success in these two cases that the decision of non-privatization was made binding, through a collective agreement in Schleswig-Holstein and municipal statute in Dresden.

Ver.di had no problem mobilizing members and allies in most of these cases; but why were some of its most multifaceted campaigns unsuccessful? Like in Britain, there was a nationwide squeeze on resources in the health system due to the DRG system being in place and insufficient investments by the states that these campaigns could not address. Local campaigners faced Conservative and Liberal politicians, at the state and municipal level, who favored privatization as the solution and, given the strong institutionalization of their role in the health system, were usually well within their rights to privatize. Their reasoning mixed expediency with the pro-market principle; in the words of a Liberal parliamentarian in Hamburg, "privatization is necessary to preserve the LBK hospitals and to preserve jobs. In addition, there is awareness that the state does not have to run hospitals. Private companies are better at it. The state only has to provide the right framework conditions" (Schinnenburg 2003). However, as the case of Dresden showed, warding off privatization under a Conservative-led local government, as well as powerful and experienced policymakers, is also possible in Germany when the campaign is not only supported by an alliance but, in addition, it is anticipatory and starts early.

5.4 Comparison

In both countries, multifaceted anti-privatization campaigns combining diverse tactics could be observed. English campaigners succeeded nearly every time, while German campaigners failed more often than they succeeded, although the former had stronger capacities to mobilize their power resources. Unexpectedly, German trade unionists took the lead in all of these campaigns, whereas English trade unionists sometimes were merely part of a campaign led by some other local group or were widely absent. These different politics reflect differences between the insurance-funded German health system and the state-dominated English system. Table 5.4 presents the main differences

Table 5.4 Trade union resources, capacities, and outcomes

		England	Germany
Resources	Membership	High	High
	Public support	Strong	Strong
	Access to decision-makers	Moderate to weak	Moderate to weak
	Legal leverage	Moderate	Moderate
Capacity	Broad framing of issues	Yes	Yes
	Sustaining local partnerships	Weak	Moderate
	Existence of and cooperation with local campaign groups	Strong	Moderate
Health system	Politics	Funding and provision politicized	Provision politicized, funding depoliticized
	Institutions	Privatizers in a weak position	Privatizers in strong position
Anti-privatization campaign outcomes		Usually success	Usually failure

Source: Own presentation.

between the two countries in terms of union resources and capacities, health system characteristics, and outcomes.

The predominance of material privatization in Germany, as opposed to outsourcing of medical services in Britain, seems to explain the difference. In Germany, unions face entire systems of municipal hospitals being transferred into the private sector, while in England the issue is particular services that are delivered in-house being purchased instead from a private provider. However, comparing the phenomenon between the two countries, other important respects are the same: privatization, whether of an asset or a function, is a for-profit takeover of health services; it has a similar policy underpinning and is opposed by campaigners for similar reasons. In both countries, trade unionists and other groups of citizens become involved in these campaigns. The form privatization takes is just one aspect of the two health systems that explains the difference in campaign outcomes.

Union resources that are emphasized in the industrial relations literature matter to some degree. Healthcare unions in both countries had strong public support (according to opinion polls), high union density (compared to overall national figures), channels of influence (through political and professional networks), and legal leverage (as could be seen in the Dresden and Bristol cases). They also have a strong capacity to frame privatization in broad policy terms beyond the interests of their members, usually stressing the value of high quality services accessible for all citizens. These common features of the two countries are important factors that distinguish healthcare unions from their counterparts in most other sectors and strengthen them in their campaigns, but they do not explain the differences between the countries.

Given other differences, the outcomes are puzzling. England's health unions have a more fragmented structure (two general unions and several occupational unions), and their local structures are usually weaker than in Germany. Ver.di, by contrast, has broad local structures covering many sectors in which staff make and maintain local political connections needed for sustained broad-based coalitions. Trade union density, in turn, is lower in Germany than in England. Nevertheless, English campaigns more effective.

Union tactics in anti-privatization campaigns matter somewhat for explaining the differences (Jalette and Hebdon 2012). Ver.di's campaign in Dresden succeeded because of a farsighted union strategy of closing off privatization as an option. English campaigners often proposed alternatives to privatization to the purchaser of services and the CCGs, which themselves were governed by medical professionals, who were sometimes receptive to their arguments. These cases of prevented privatization might have ended differently in the absence of multifaceted campaigns and strong grassroots campaign groups.

However, a combination of multiple tactics by unions was neither a necessary nor a sufficient condition for success. Some successful English campaigns were not even led by unions: they were led by grassroots groups such as PoN, and their outcomes cannot be attributed to union strategy. In addition, some of ver.di's tactically sophisticated campaigns did not stop privatization. At LBK Hamburg, the mobilization of members and allies, the framing of the issue as a health system and democracy issue and the use of the ballot initiative could be observed. This was after a long history of working as comanagers on alternatives to privatization and was followed with negotiations over the effects. At Marburg-Gießen, ver.di participated in both a coalition with local civil society and a planning commission by the Conservative state government. These two highly sophisticated German campaigns failed to stop privatization.

The likelihood of a campaign's success seems to depend on varying marketization conditions that can be expected to matter in healthcare more generally: the politicization and funding of healthcare, and the organizational basis of privatizers.

First, state domination of the NHS created conditions for a much higher degree of politicization than the mixed economy of German healthcare. This political constraint could be seen in the mobilization against the 2012 Act and its continuation afterward, in a series of uncoordinated campaigns against privatization that shaped the agenda of the 2015 general election. Local commissioning exercises in England were framed as a threat to the integrity of the national system, and Conservative policymakers had to distance themselves from privatization. Unions, but also grassroots campaign groups, recognized and used this political opportunity. In Germany, by contrast, competition and ownership were separate matters – the one handled in national laws and the other handled in a series of much more contentious local decisions – and campaigners had little recourse to address market pressures cited as reasons for privatization. Although Germans generally support public sector healthcare provision, ver.di's *Gesundheitskampagne* shows the difficulty of reforming the health system in a way that addresses the proximate causes of privatization.

Second, key decision-makers in the NHS were more susceptible to pressure from campaigners and their decisions more readily reversible than their counterparts in German state and local government. These organizational constraints can be attributed to the CCGs' lack of experience and the complex regulatory mechanics governing purchasing. The resulting uncertainty – compounded by downward pressure on prices due to years of in-house wage restraint in the NHS that made public sector providers highly competitive in tendering exercises – is a reason why private players were withdrawing for commercial reasons, from contracts (Hinchingbrooke) and commissioning exercises (West Sussex). Privatization decisions in Germany, by contrast, were made by local politicians, with functions underpinned by a written constitution and electoral mandate. Moreover, there were no cases of reversing material privatization, in part because of the expense of buying back hospitals.

5.5 Conclusion

In this chapter, the conditions of success and failure in campaigns to protect public healthcare services were explored. The outcomes of these campaigns depended mainly on the differences between the marketization processes brought about by the social insurance and national health systems and their corresponding salience. While there were strong multifaceted campaigns contesting privatization in both systems, in the state-dominated English system these campaigns also led to the politicization of the market and the collapse of privatization efforts. English anti-privatization campaigns were thus more effective.

The findings highlight the importance of sector-specific marketization processes and the corresponding political opportunities that can vary internationally, but produce outcomes that are the opposite of what theory would predict. As Table 5.4 shows, unions in both countries had strong resources for campaigning. Nevertheless, English campaigns tended to be more successful than German ones. This can be explained with constraints that marketization in the state-dominated NHS imposes for privatizers and political opportunities for campaigners that are not present in the insurance-funded German health system. The evidence on market-making leading to new union strategies in German healthcare is similar to other sectors, including privatized and outsourced telecommunications (e.g., Doellgast 2012), temporary agencies in the automotive sector (e.g., Benassi and Dorigatti 2015), and internationalized networks of construction contractors (e.g., Greer, Ciupijus, and Lillie 2013). In the context of health systems, and possibly public services more generally, the politicization and funding of services, the organizational vulnerabilities of decision-makers, as well as the existence of and cooperation with grassroots campaign groups seem to shape campaign outcomes.

While campaign outcomes could be explained, it remains open, why German unions took the lead in all the campaigns, while English unions missed the chance and merely participated in many of the campaigns, which were led by others. One possible explanation might be that German unions possess stronger local structures or that healthcare is more politicized in England in general, leading to less of a need for union leadership.

Since privatization of medical services is the most recent form of marketization and the marketization process is still ongoing, the findings are only valid in the time context under study. The successful German anti-privatization campaign in the case of Dresden showed that unions in Germany can overcome the strong institutional role of local policymakers and lower politicization of private provision of health services. German trade unionists might learn from this case to influence the rules of the healthcare market, to take all forms of marketization into account and anticipate their facilitating function for further marketization. Furthermore, an extension of networking from mainly parties to grassroots initiatives, as in the English cases, might grant them additional societal power and repertoires of contention. In the same way, over time, English purchasers of health services may learn how to push through large-scale privatization of health services, as the latest Virgin Health contract might suggest.

Note

1. There are, however, examples of commissioning processes of values below £50m that moved forward. This includes community health services in Essex (2015), which were handed to a social enterprise; community health services in Surrey (2012) and children's health services in Wiltshire and Devon, which have been taken over by Virgin Care (2015); and prison health services in London, which have been taken over by Care UK (2016). Numerous smaller contracts taken by these and other firms could be named as well. But these are all cases where there was no opposition from unions.

References

Augener, Manfred. 2009. Bürgerbegehren ist schon angelaufen. *Hamburger Abendblatt.* http://www.abendblatt.de/region/pinneberg/article107530368/Buergerbegehren-ist-schon-angelaufen.html.

Baggott, Rob. 2004. *Health and Health Care in Britain.* 3rd edition. Basingstoke: Macmillan Education.

BBC. 2013. George Eliot Hospital Takeover Plans Approved by Government. *BBC News. 5 September.* http://www.bbc.com/news/uk-england-coventry-warwickshire-23968538.

BBC. 2014. Staffordshire Cancer Care 'Could Be Privatised'. *BBC News. 3 July.* http://www.bbc.com/news/uk-england-stoke-staffordshire-28144161.

BBC. 2015. Staffordshire Cancer Petition Handed to NHS Bosses. *BBC News. 4 June.* http://www.bbc.com/news/uk-england-stoke-staffordshire-33014991.

BBC. 2016. Staffordshire £1.2bn Cancer Contract Given Green Light. https://www.bbc.com/news/uk-england-stoke-staffordshire-38115713.

Benassi, Chiara, and Lisa Dorigatti. 2015. Straight to the Core: Explaining Union Responses to the Casualization of Work: the IG Metall Campaign for Agency Workers. *British Journal of Industrial Relations* no. 53 (3):533–555.

Cameron, Amanda. 2016. Virgin Care Wins £700m Contract to Run Health and Care Services in Bath and North East Somerset. *Bath Chronicle, November 10, 2016.* https://www.bathchronicle.co.uk/news/health/virgin-care-wins-700m-contract-223150.

Doellgast, Virginia. 2012. *Disintegrating Democracy at Work.* Ithaca: Cornell University Press.

Express & Star. 2015. £1.2bn Bid to Privatise Cancer and End-Of-Life Care in Staffordshire rejected. *Express & Star, 15 October.* http://www.expressandstar.com/news/2015/10/15/1-2bn-bid-to-privatise-cancer-and-end-of-life-care-in-staffordshire-rejected/.

Foster, Deborah, and Peter Scott. 1998. Conceptualising Union Responses to Contracting Out Municipal Services, 1979–97. *Industrial Relations Journal* no. 29 (2):137–150.

Glassner, Vera, Susanne Pernicka, and Nele Dittmar. 2015. *Arbeitsbeziehungen im Krankenhaussektor, Project Report.* Linz: University of Linz.

Greer, Ian. 2008. Social Movement Unionism and Social Partnership in Germany: The Case of Hamburg's Hospitals. *Industrial Relations* no. 47 (4):602–624.

Greer, Ian, Thorsten Schulten, and Nils Böhlke. 2013. How Does Market Making affect Industrial Relations? Evidence from Eight German Hospitals. *British Journal of Industrial Relations* no. 51 (2):215–239.

Greer, Ian, Zinovijus Ciupijus, and Nathan Lillie. 2013. The European Migrant Workers Union and the Barriers to Transnational Industrial Citizenship. *European Journal of Industrial Relations* no. 19 (1):5–20.

Halbwachs, Maurice. 1985. *Das Gedächtnis und seme sozialen Bedingungen*. Berlin: Suhrkamp.

Hill, Matthew. 2014. Legal Challenge over NHS Spending. *BBC News. 2 May*. http://www.bbc.com/news/health-27239242

Hood, Alice. 2011. All Together for the NHS. 15 March. http://touchstoneblog.org.uk/2011/03/all-together-for-the-nhs/.

Mori, Ipsos. 2015. Coming to Terms with Austerity? 28 October. https://www.ipsos-mori.com/researchpublications/researcharchive/3644/Coming-to-terms-with-austerity.aspx.

Jalette, Patrice, and Robert Hebdon. 2012. Unions and Privatization: Opening the "Black box". *Industrial & Labor Relations Review* no. 65 (1):17–35.

Jenkins, Lin. 2014. NHS 'People's March' Campaigners Arrive in London after 300-Mile March. *The Guardian. 6 September*. http://www.theguardian.com/society/2014/sep/06/nhs-future-darlo-mums-protest-march-london.

Kolarczyk, Arne. 2009. Bürgerbegehren zum Klinik-Verkauf gescheitert. *Hamburger Abendblatt, August 5*. http://www.abendblatt.de/region/pinneberg/article107541217/Buergerbegehren-zum-Klinik-Verkauf-gescheitert.html

Leng, Freya. 2014. UnitingCare Partnership Chosen as Preferred Bidder for Cambridgeshire's Older People's Healthcare Contract. *Cambridge News. 1 October*. http://www.cambridge-news.co.uk/UnitingCare-Partnership-chosen-preferred-bidder/story-23025347-detail/story.html

Malyon, Mike. 2015. Miliband Applauds Nuneaton Hospital's Vision for 'Integrated Health and Social Care'. *Coventry Telegraph. 26 January*. http://www.coventrytelegraph.net/news/local-news/milliband-appluads-nuneaton-hospitals-shared-8520267.

NHS. 2017. Transforming Cancer and End of Life Care Programme. https://www.staffordsurroundsccg.nhs.uk/our-services2/cancer-and-end-of-life-care.

PoN. 2014. Some Facts about What Happened to Our NHS. https://protectournhs.files.wordpress.com/2014/11/some-facts-about-whats-happened-to-our-nhs-nov-2014.pdf.

Robinson, Nick. 2014. Miliband Promises to Make NHS Priority. *BBC News. 12 May*. http://www.bbc.com/news/uk-politics-27385204.

RP Online. 2007. Klinik-Verkauf: Verdi für Kooperation. http://www.rp-online.de/nrw/staedte/krefeld/klinik-verkauf-verdi-fuer-kooperation-aid-1.648495.

Ryan, Siobhan. 2015. Bupa CSH Pulls Out of West Sussex MSK Contract Negotiations. *Daily Echo. 26 January*. http://www.dailyecho.co.uk/news/11749292.Bupa_CSH_pulls_out_of_West_Sussex_MSK_contract_negotiations/.

Schinnenburg, Wieland. 2003. Speech in the Bürgerschaft der Freien und Hansestadt Hamburg. *17th Parliamentary Term, 51st Session. Plenary Transcript 17/51, November 26th*.

Siebelt, Frank. 2013. Fresenius wird größter Klinikbetreiber Europas. *Manager-Magazin. 13 September*. http://www.manager-magazin.de/unternehmen/artikel/kauf-von-rhoen-kliniken-fresenius-wird-groesster-klinikbetreiber-europas-a-922014.html.

Stretton, Rachel. 2014. UPDATE: Campaigners Welcome 'Courageous' Decision by Hospital Bosses to Keep Pathology Service. *Dorset Echo. 8 October*. http://www.dorsetecho.co.uk/news/11522207.UPDATE__Campaigners_welcome__courageous__decision_by_hospital_bosses_to_keep_pathology_service/.

Swinford, Steven. 2015. Ed Miliband Said He Wanted to 'Weaponise' NHS in Secret Meeting with BBC Executives. *The Guardian. 11 January*. http://www.telegraph.co.uk/news/politics/ed-miliband/11338695/Ed-Miliband-said-he-wanted-to-weaponise-NHS-in-secret-meeting-with-BBC-executives.html.

The Times. 2011. NHS Reform Is a 'Potential Disaster. *The Times. January 17.* http://www.thetimes.co.uk/tto/opinion/letters/article2876573.ece.

TUC. 2011. All Together for the NHS – The Campaign. 9 June. https://www.tuc.org.uk/industrial-issues/all-together-nhs/all-together-nhs-campaign.

UNISON. 2013. 999 – Answer the Call for Your NHS. https://www.unison.org.uk/our-campaigns/999-answer-the-call-for-your-nhs/.

UNISON. 2014a. Bidders Shortlist for Cancer and End of Life Care Contracts in Staffordshire Is Alarming Says UNISON. 6 November. https://www.unison.org.uk/news/article/2014/11/bidders-shortlist-for-cancer-and-end-of-life-care-contracts-in-staffordshire-is-alarming-says-unison/.

UNISON. 2014b. UNISON Victory over Weston General Hospital Privatisation Threat. 4 June. https://www.unison.org.uk/news/article/2014/06/unison-victory-over-weston-general-hospital-privatisation-threat/.

UNISON. 2016. Suspension of Planned Privatisation of Cancer Services in Staffs. https://www.unison.org.uk/news/press-release/2016/02/suspension-of-planned-privatisation-of-cancer-services-in-staffs-welcomed-by-unison/.

UNITE. 2014. George Eliot Hospital Is at a Crossroads. http://www.unitetheunion.org/uploaded/documents/6303_GEH_A5_Flayer_211-16328.pdf.

ver.di. 2003. *Aus: wertung Gesundheitskampgne – Erkentnisse und Erfahrungen zur Kampagnenarbeit in ver.di.* Berlin: ver.di.

Wright, Tom. 2014. MP Pleased with Hospital's NHS Ruling. *Weston Mercury.* 6 June. http://www.thewestonmercury.co.uk/news/mp_pleased_with_hospital_s_nhs_ruling_1_3629718.

Wulff, Herbert. 2005. Die Patientenversorgung leidet. *Junge Welt. 29 November.* https://www.jungewelt.de/loginFailed.php?ref=/2005/11-29/024.php.

6 Reversing marketization effects[*]

Mobilizing workers and the public for staffing levels

6.1 Introduction

Measures to increase productivity and competition that led to marketization and privatization had considerable effects on workers and patients. Increased efficiency, i.e., a rising number of patients treated in shorter times, came at a cost for hospital staff and, most pronounced, for nurses. They experienced an increase in the intensity of their work (Clark et al. 2001; Lafer 2005; Moody 2014). As a consequence, not only morale among nurses dropped and dissatisfaction grew (Aiken et al. 2013) but also care-related mistakes and risks for complications increased. Research clearly indicates a strong association between inappropriate workloads for nurses and worse health outcomes (see, e.g., Kane et al. 2007; Aiken et al. 2011; Cook et al. 2012; Schreyögg 2016). In this way, and to give one of the most drastic examples, an increase in nurses' workload by one patient increases the likelihood of an inpatient dying within 30 days of admission by 7 per cent (Aiken et al. 2014). Patient and nurse outcomes are consistently better in hospitals with better staffing levels. Patients in the hospitals with the highest patient-to-nurse ratios in England had 26 per cent higher mortality rates. Furthermore, nurses in those hospitals were twice as likely to be dissatisfied with their jobs, showed high burnout levels and reported low or deteriorating quality of care (Rafferty et al. 2007). Poor staffing also leads to working overtime, which is associated with reports of poor or failing patient safety, poor quality of care, and more care being left undone (Ausserhofer et al. 2013; Griffiths et al. 2014).

In this complex of issues, trade unions can protect not only workers but also patients by achieving better working conditions. For example, one cross-sectional study showed 5.7 per cent lower mortality rates for hospitals with nurse unions (Seago and Ash 2002), and another showed significant decreases in hospital-acquired illnesses in unionized hospitals (Dube, Kaplan, and Thompson 2016). While unions' regulation of staffing levels may underlie these findings, it

[*] The German and US American case studies are the result of joint research with Nick Krachler, Cornell University, School of Industrial and Labor Relations, njk77@cornell.edu. Parts of this research have also been published as journal article (Auffenberg and Krachler 2017).

is unclear under which conditions unions can achieve this objective. In healthcare, the fact that nurse associations globally have identified staffing levels as their first priority and still have had uneven success in regulating staffing (Clark and Clark 2003) indicates that what is needed is a further understanding of the conditions under which these endeavours can be successful.

One possibility to take staffing and wage costs partly out of competition are statutory or collectively agreed patient-to-staff ratios. Nurse unions are facing particular difficulties but also chances in their work emanating from nurses' professional ethos and the fact that strikes can potentially put patients at risk. There are three general strategies to deal with these challenges. (1) Healthcare or nurse unions can employ professionalism as a strategy (Gordon 2009). This entails a strict no-strike policy, a focus on providing nurses with educational opportunities and lobbying politicians with research reports. The Royal College of Nursing (RCN) in England has pursued this strategy, leading to divisions among English nurse unions and weakening their bargaining power (Jennings and Western 1997). (2) Another strategy is militancy, in particular through the use of strikes (Briskin 2012). This strategy is designed to bring managers to the negotiating table, traditionally for the purposes of negotiating higher wages. In the context of professionals such as nurses, this strategy may be problematic if it contradicts professional norms. The potential negative effect of increasing mortality rates through nurse strikes (Gruber and Kleiner 2012) feeds into nurses' aversion to using the strike as the only strategy. (3) To avoid the problems named with professionalism and militancy, US nurse unions have developed a "craft-professional hybrid model" (Ash, Seago, and Spetz 2014, 396) that combines collective bargaining with mobilization through professional norms and practices. The Minnesota Nurses Association, the California Nurses Association and the Service Employees International Union (SEIU) have employed a dual strategy of regulating patient care through collective bargaining agreements, as well as through public and legislative campaigns. The California Nurses Association has had the most success, achieving a law mandating minimum staffing levels across the State in 1999 (Clark and Clark 2006). While this strategy was successful in California, previous research does not clarify why it has not led to more success in other states and whether this strategy can also be successful in other national institutional configurations.

Faced with the same pressures for efficiency and work intensification, trade unions in all three countries studied in this chapter – Germany, England and the USA – have been struggling for higher staffing levels in the mid-2010s. Nevertheless, their strategies to achieve this aim differed. The biggest trade union in the German hospital sector, ver.di, pursued this aim at the national level, by campaigning and lobbying for statutory staffing levels. This approach was influence-driven and characterized by cooperation and the provision of expertise. At the same time, ver.di pursued the introduction of mandatory staffing levels at the local level, through agreements with the employer. The approach at this level is more membership-driven and draws on confrontational and militant measures. The biggest nursing trade unions in England pursued a joint national lobbying strategy, but lacked strong complementary and confrontational local-level activism. Besides different structural features of the trade unions in the two countries, interviews with German and English trade unionists suggest that this difference might be explained with different framing processes. While German trade unionists expressed fundamental criticism of the reimbursement system, a strong professional ethos and self-concept as non-militant unions impeded taking more confrontational action in England. Due to its striking parallels and differing from other empirical chapters of this book, this chapter features a third case from the US. It follows the logic of case comparison of the previous chapters and aims at widening the understanding why nurse unions in the USA and Germany have adopted similar strategies – with success – despite different national institutions. Like ver.di, the New York State Nurses Association (NYSNA) adopted a dual strategy of regulating staffing levels through collective bargaining agreements that were achieved following a combined strategy of organizing and social movement unionism, as well as public legislative campaigns. The same factors have enabled unions in very different national industrial relations and healthcare systems to adopt the same strategies.

In this chapter, it will be argued that unions can adopt successful strategies if they can leverage or enhance the sources of power their proximate, local contexts afford them. While broader political economy trends, like marketization, may create common problems unions should respond to, only those unions that draw on opportunity structures to transform their organizational structures, mobilize resources such as the media, politicians, community members, and local activist networks, and that frame issues as broad sociopolitical problems, calling on a society- or class-based identity of empowerment to mobilize members, are likely to successfully employ activist strategies.

After briefly having discussed the obstacles specific to trade unionism in the nursing profession, this chapter will give general information on the cases studied and present the findings. To conclude, findings will be compared and the limitations as well as the implications for trade union strategy will be considered.

6.2 Information on understaffing cases

The three case studies are embedded in two most-different systems designs. Cases in this chapter are defined as trade union strategies designed to combat understaffing, i.e., inadequate levels of registered nurse staffing that may undermine patient safety. Success in this chapter is defined as the achievement of mandatory and enforceable staffing levels, either statutory or laid down in a collective agreement. The English respectively US American cases are most different from the German case regarding their welfare state, healthcare system, and employment relations contexts. Based on this national-level setting, one would expect trade unions to be confronted with different challenges and, accordingly, to pursue different goals and choose different strategies. Actors in all countries pursued the goal of improving staffing levels. The English case differs from the German one since the English union pursued a partnership strategy whereas the German and US American case studies are similar in their outcome of a combined social movement and organizing strategy (for more information on research design and methods see Chapter 1).

Like Britain, the USA have a liberal welfare state and less-coordinated employment relations in a liberal market economy, however, with a private insurance-based healthcare system. In this setting, trade unions would not be expected to be confronted with similar challenges as in Germany and to pursue the same goals using comparable strategies, and be successful with it. Both trade unions pursued the same goal (regulation of safe staffing levels) and used very similar strategies to attain these (a mix of collective bargaining that included coalition-building and organizing at the workplace level, as well as public legislative campaigns at the national level). This is particularly surprising for Germany, in which unions would be expected to draw on their institutional resources and exert influence predominantly through institutional coordination at the national sector level.

Through the case selection, some possible sources of variation were reduced. All trade unions represent nurses or, respectively, that part of the national trade union that represents nurses. Furthermore, because the same period of time is analyzed (from the mid-2000s to the end of April 2016 with a peak in activity between 2012/13 and 2016), time-variant factors, such as the international economic and financial situation, can be ruled out as possible explanations. The settings of London, Berlin, and New York are all large, metropolitan, and politically and economically highly important regions.

Regarding data generation, interviews were conducted with trade union leaders, workplace representatives, and activists. The case studies are based on five interviews for England, seven interviews (including one focus group interview with five participants) for Germany, and twelve interviews for New York State (quotes from interviews are marked as "IP"). The interview data was triangulated with an analysis of around 50 documents, including trade union policy documents, government reports, press releases, videos, collective bargaining agreements, newspaper articles, and various outputs from social media outlets.

6.3 Trade union responses to understaffing

The three cases will first be presented separately, following a common structure to increase comparability. Finally, the cases will be compared in the last part of this section.

6.3.1 Findings: England

In England, the issue of understaffing was targeted mostly at the national level, but also at the local level, and by several actors. Both main unions in which nurses are organized, the RCN and UNISON, worked on the issue of staffing levels. These two – usually competing – unions were pursuing slightly different approaches, but also cooperating in the Safe Staffing Alliance (SSA). While the RCN has been lobbying for staffing levels for decades, UNISON's Be Safe campaign and the SSA were initiated following the Mid-Staffordshire scandal in 2008–2009 that became salient again in 2013 through publication of the inquiry into the scandal in the Francis Report and a general inquiry on care quality of 13more foundation trusts in the Keogh Report (Francis 2013; Keogh 2013). These reports stirred considerable public concern about deficient hospital hygiene and care quality that were attributed to cost pressures and insufficient staffing levels.

The SSA was founded in response to the publication of the Francis and Keogh Reports – not by the unions, but by the Patients Association (PA) in 2013 (IP16: 2–46). The membership bodies of the SSA were UNISON, the RCN, the PA, the Nursing Standard (a newspaper), the Florence Nightingale Foundation and several individuals, such as directors and academics specialized in nursing, independent nurses in the private sector and management consultants (IP16: 10–66). The first activity of the SSA was to collate, through a care campaign, evidence on registered nurse numbers and the impact on patient care outcomes (IP16: 2–46). The RCN responded in a similar way to the Francis inquiry, stressing the point of insufficient staffing in addition to a complex interaction of several factors, such as finance, culture, bullying, and lack of whistleblowing (IP01: 4–65). UNISON responded in a different way from the RCN, complementing lobbying activities pursued within the SSA framework with a workplace campaign. The UNISON Be Safe campaign was also set up in response to the Francis and Keogh Reports and it aimed at normalizing the complaints procedure; at making it easier for staff to raise concerns about their work setting, patient safety, staff safety and equipment. The campaign also addressed the employers with a training program that would help employers regard these concerns as "golden nuggets of information and encourage them to pause, to reflect, and see what needs to be done differently" (IP02: 2–64). The campaign did not exceed the stage of pilot projects that were only carried out in trusts in which the employers approved UNISON to carry out their campaign (IP02: 6).

6.3.1.1 Resources and capabilities

The SSA drew its strength mostly from societal power, i.e., public support, good access to the media, and prestige of its members, while almost completely neglecting organizational power that could have been activated by mobilizing nurses. In its Be Safe workplace campaign, UNISON seemed to rely on institutional power, trying to cooperatively carry out their campaign only where employers agreed to it, matching their market-oriented identity. Accordingly, UNISON also left the organizational power of nurses widely unused.

The national staffing levels campaign of the SSA could benefit from strong societal power stemming from public support and good access to the media. The alliance recognized and used this power to their own benefit. Especially after reports raised considerable concerns about care quality, the topic received strong public attention, especially since the Keogh Report revealed that the situation had not improved eight years after the Francis Report was issued (IP16: 8–64). Also for the work in the years to follow these reports, the chair of the SSA felt that "[the] public [was] fueling the quality regulator" (IP16: 9–60) because "[the] NHS is cherished; if the government starts to break it down and doesn't fund it properly, there is an outcry by the UK public, for its health service" (IP16: 6–59). The SSA also further benefited from high public support because of the credibility of their members (IP16: 10–66). Especially the Patients' Association gave leverage to public support, particularly with their president Sir Robert Francis, author of the report of the same name (IP16: 6–59).

One of the key recommendations of the Francis Report was the establishment of guidelines for staffing levels that resulted in the National Institute for Health and Care Excellence (NICE) guidance. These guidelines were suspended by the NHS England chief executive in 2015, which gave another boost to the supporters of safe staffing levels. According to the SSA, "the public were really up in arms" (IP16: 8–44) when NICE was suspended, also because it had cost about £20m. This "political faux pas" (IP16: 8–44) and the consequent media attention were used by the parties of the SSA to promote their cause through an open letter that was sent to the newspapers and received good media coverage (IP16: 10–68).

Related to the aforementioned high public interest for care quality, the access to media, leveraged through the SSA, was "very good" (IP16: 7–56). The SSA was quoted in national newspapers because journalists appreciated the sensible and evidence-based information (IP16: 10–66). The fact that a newspaper, the Nursing Standard, was one of the SSA's members, additionally increased their coverage in the media since other newspapers picked up articles published in the Nursing Standard (IP16: 1–66). The allies of the SSA seemed to know how to benefit from the public's interest in care quality and the salience of the topic. They also provided scientific evidence that supported the relation between high staffing levels and good care quality. However, the SSA did not use a mobilizing frame that referred to the public interest of good care quality, but restricted itself to a rather technical argumentation. The SSA showed a society-orientated identity and regarded itself as a promoter of staffing levels and a provider of relevant expertise.

Based on the aforementioned good reputation of its five member organizations and its individual members holding positions in politics, the SSA also had good access to decision makers (IP16: 10–66) (Safe Staffing Alliance 2017). They lobbied the House of Lords and the House of Commons, so that members of parliament (MPs) supported their cause (IP16: 7–59).

A resource the SSA could have potentially drawn additional strength from, but did not succeed to activate, were frontline nurses. Even though the SSA put up a website on which employees could log their concerns if they were working in unsafe areas, and the chair of the SSA would council them on how to take action, this tool was barely used. Therefore, the chair admitted that the SSA needed to revitalize this part of its activities and get more nurses engaged (IP16: 12–64).

Unions in England struggled with the mobilization of nurses, too. The uses of associational or organizational power were impaired by the competitive relationship between the RCN and UNISON. This disadvantage of a fragmented union structure was overcome in parts through cooperation between UNISON and the RCN in the SSA. However, the cooperation had its limits: "We [UNISON and the RCN] are as joined up as we can be, but the other thing is we are both competing against each other" (IP08: 14–62). In this way, both unions also pursued their own additional, separate safe staffing campaigns and advocated different positions regarding mandatory staffing levels. The SSA thus did not have a clear and unified stance on whether it supported mandatory staffing levels or non-binding staffing guidelines (IP16: 3–58, IP08: 13–59, IP01: 6–54).

In their workplace campaign, UNISON could benefit from associational power arising from unusual cooperation of the different levels. The Be Safe campaign was coordinated by their national head of nursing and implemented locally (IP08: 9–65). However, a local-level trade unionist and nurse responsible for the campaign in his trust complained about a lack of human resources: "I get three days a week facility time and I don't get any additional time to do the nursing thing" (IP08: 4–56). This could not be compensated by support of active members despite a high union density of 50 to 60 per cent in the respective pilot trust. Communication with members, especially nurses, was considered difficult: "The biggest issue is most nurses don't bother reading their e-mails, unfortunately. They don't have time and they go home and they don't really want to read e-mails from work-type things" (IP08: 3–61). Other means of communication, such as social media or telephone campaigning, were not mentioned.

Therefore, UNISON did not manage to mobilize their members sufficiently, which can possibly also be traced back to their market-orientation and the pursuit of business unionism and partnership. They only started their campaign in trusts in which employers agreed with it and were willing to participate in safe staffing trainings. Moreover, UNISON did not use an empowerment or mobilization frame in this matter, but, on the contrary, the London head of nursing working in one of the pilot trusts doubted the potential of mobilization among their nurse members:

> [Nurses] join a union, they want peace of mind that if something goes wrong, they've got protection. If they make a mistake at work or someone accuses them of something, they'll have representation. If their job comes under threat the union will come and support them but other than that they don't really to a greater extent want to involve themselves in the union.
> —(IP08: 4–48).

Nevertheless, the aim of the UNISON Be Safe campaign was to empower nurses. At least theoretically, and promoted by the national level, UNISON wanted to train nurses, increase their confidence and encourage them to raise concerns. Furthermore, the national head of nursing stated that she thought that in the past, nurses were "sometimes worried about rocking the boat" (IP02: 3–69). The training was therefore built on convincing nurses that they have a right to raise a concern, to be listened to and to be believed, and to have their concerns acted upon (IP02: 3–69). Nonetheless, UNISON did not even succeed at motivating nurses to fill out the Be Safe forms following the trainings (IP08: 6–57). Ironically, a lack of time also kept staff from filling out the forms. A UNISON local trade unionist reported that before nursing staff numbers were increased in 2015, nurses were constantly short of staff, and they basically would have to fill out an incident form every single shift. Moreover, local managers discouraged employees from using them, because it would reflect badly on them and the hospital's reputation. Senior managers accepted it as a legitimate use of the employer's system, though (IP08: 5–47).

In contrast to UNISON, RCN recognized staffing levels as a good topic for mobilization:

> The one [thing nurses] always say is most important to them, […] is the ability to use their clinical expertise, their knowledge, their training, to the best effect and to be allowed to deliver and use that care in a safe environment where they can treat patients in a safe way.
>
> —(IP01: 4–53)

Furthermore, as the RCN national policy advisor added, it is a topic that could mobilize nurses who usually would not strike (IP01: 6–53):

> The one thing they say they're prepared to strike [about] is not actually about pay, it's actually about safety of their own patients. […] that's the one that stresses them out […] that gets them down and ill. It's the whole factor about them not being able to deliver safe and effective outcomes for their patients.
>
> —(IP01: 6–61)[1]

Therefore, the RCN expressly used this topic for mobilization: "This is why it always comes into our key messages whatever we talk about, whichever way we go" (IP01: 6–61). Nevertheless, the RCN did not report any of its own workplace activism or other mobilization of its members.

6.3.1.2 Strategies

Matching the resources of strong public interest in good care quality and the advantageous access to the media and to some policymakers, the SSA mainly pursued a strategy of lobbying and influencing the public discourse at the national level. UNISON, in turn, pursued a workplace partnership strategy that lacked a strong institutional power basis. The RCN meanwhile focused on professionalism and lobbying.

Based on its strong societal power resources, the SSA's main strategies were placing the issue of staffing levels in the media and lobbying policymakers. The SSA described itself as a pressure or campaigning group (IP16: 1–66). As mentioned above, the PA with their president Sir Robert Francis, who examined the Mid-Staffordshire hospital services, founded the SSA (IP16: 2–57). It is noteworthy that it was not the trade unions who took the initiative, but, as was shown in the previous chapter on the anti-privatization campaigns, trade unions in England again left the initiative to other civil society or grassroots organizations (IP16: 10–68).

Although part of the same alliance, the single members seemed to mostly work independently from one another. As the head of the SSA described it: "UNISON are doing an awful lot, lobbying their members as well, linking in with MPs, the Commons and in the House of Lords, as is the RCN" (IP16: 11–69).

The SSA recognized staffing levels as a topic of both the public and the nurses' interest (IP01: 9–62). However, there were no efforts undertaken to mobilize nurses (besides a form on the internet that nurses could use to file complaints that was barely used) or other allies. Joint action of the SSA was widely restricted to "keeping the whole notion of safe staffing alive" (IP16: 10–68) by intervening in the public discourse, publishing articles in the Nursing Standards, giving interviews and posing questions to healthcare organizations (IP16: 10–68). The SSA also kept the topic on the agenda by providing and spreading evidence. As the national RCN trade unionists explained, "the whole rationale of that group [the SSA] is to say here is the evidence" (IP01: 6–56). The SSA restricted its activity to the promotion and dissemination of scientific studies on staffing levels (IP16: 5–68, 6–60) without taking a clear stance.

A coherent, own strategy for the alliance, as well as clear demands, seemed to be lacking. There was no unity with regards to the aims among the five members of the SSA. Their head stated that the alliance was separated into two groups: one that supported mandated staffing levels, similar to those in California or Australia, and another group that was worried about setting staffing levels because it would be difficult to change them again, and argued that such levels would not be funded anyway (IP16: 3–59). The only demand the five members of the alliance agreed upon was that one nurse should never be responsible for more than eight patients (IP01: 7–51).

The RCN clearly rejected mandatory staffing levels and strongly supported the suspended NICE system, lobbying for its re-introduction instead. The Care Quality Commission, responsible for examining the compliance with NICE guidance, repeatedly identified staffing levels as a source of quality problems. However, the NICE guidance neither defined concrete staffing levels for wards nor did it include sanctions (IP01: 10–49). The NICE guidance was also supported by the RCN, since it served as a possibility for it to improve its role in partnership as they were usually asked for their input in the inspections (IP01: 11–63).

Furthermore, UNISON did not clearly demand ratios at that time (IP17: 25), since "no size fits all", and "because they can work against you as well as for you".

In addition, there was a skepticism toward nurses: "The problem is sometimes you have got higher levels of staff and people take their feet off the accelerators" (IP08: 13–59, 14–59).

Another pillar of the SSA's work were lobbying efforts. Some members of the House of Lords are members or supporters of the alliance (IP16: 1–51), and the SSA's members linked with the MPs and ministers, put down questions and advanced initiatives in the House of Lords and House of Commons, as well as collected signatures for a manifesto (IP16: 7–59). However, the lobbying of decision makers was perceived as requiring patience and stamina: "it's slow, you have to wait for a crisis before you really get something to bite" (IP16: 7–59). Not surprisingly, and in accordance with its main objective of fostering the public discourse on staffing levels, the SSA was satisfied that it put the topic on the agenda and succeeded in keeping it alive. The alliance regarded this as its main achievement (IP16: 4–66).

UNISON complemented the national level actions as member of the SSA with its workplace-level Be Safe campaign that was not directly linked to a national campaign or the SSA. The aim was to normalize work overload complaints by encouraging employees, but also training management (IP08: 9–63). Convincing members to fill out the Be Safe forms was difficult because the notifications remained without any consequences (IP08: 5–47). To get members involved, UNISON initially wanted to train and empower nurses to speak up. In the end, only the Be Safe forms were distributed and only a few pilot trainings performed where the employer approved them. Trade unionists only talked to one or two key people on the ward about what to do with the forms when they were distributed instead of teaching about their use in a proper classroom session to enable nurses to fill out forms independently or as a whole ward (IP08: 6–57, 7–61). This appears to have decreased the potential for mobilization, since there was an idea of organizing beyond these trainings: "if we start getting people coming in to these drop-in training sessions [they might] get more active [...]. They'll get the organizing angle and they might actually want to take on some work themselves" (IP08: 8–39). The trainings, initially planned for the end of 2014, were put on hold during the pay dispute: "The forms were there, they were very much left to activists in workplaces to use them or not use them. And that's why, I think, to a greater or lesser extent, it's a great idea but flawed in that respect" (IP08: 7–61).

6.3.1.3 Outcome

The SSA, with its focus on lobbying, provision of expertise and influencing the public discussion, managed to repeatedly set the topic of safe staffing levels on the agenda of the public and Parliament. The number of staff was increased as a result of the care quality scandals and the safe staffing campaigns (RCN 2014, 15), but regulations on staffing levels are still missing. On the contrary, the NICE guidance was suspended in 2015. The lack of a clear and unified demand for mandatory or voluntary staffing levels probably weakened the SSA's impact on politics.

The evaluation of the Be Safe campaign's success was mixed. In light of the little use of the Be Safe forms and flawed implementation of the idea of trainings, it was evaluated as rather unsuccessful. In the opinion of a workplace trade union representative and nurse, the campaign remained below its full potential and did not reach the grassroots of the organization (IP08: 9–63). The problem was that trade unionists were continuously dealing with too many conflicts: "you could probably have a campaign every week [...]. Everyone is too busy firefighting in this country" (IP08: 9–63), for instance, with regards to mergers and acquisitions of hospitals at that time (IP08: 9–63). Finally, the Be Safe campaign was not continued. It is debatable why there was no campaign participation in the workplaces. Even though UNISON recognized the opportunity of the public pressure on management created by the Mid-Staffordshire scandal and had very similar ideas to ver.di in Berlin to use it to its own benefit, it did not ultimately have any effect. This might be due to the framing of the issue solely in terms of employment relations and not in the wider societal issue terms. In addition, UNISON appeared to doubt their own mobilization capacities and the power of nurses. This might have worked as a self-fulfilling prophecy. There was also some suspicion that nurses would slow down their work if staffing was improved. Last, but not least, the partnership approach lacked a sanctions mechanism and was based merely on the goodwill of employers. The lack of personnel resources appeared to be a problem as well.

The RCN showed a more positive attitude toward their members and nurses. The union recognized the issue of understaffing as a main concern of nurses, but did not engage in workplace activities to mobilize employees.

Unused resources and the choice of strategies that only in part matched those resources seem to explain the limited success of unions and the alliance in this matter. Resources that were present in England, such as the strong associational power, were not used by UNISON for its campaign. Neither did UNISON use the societal power resource of the SSA or promote other networks for their purposes. The SSA itself did not agree upon common demands regarding safe staffing. UNISON's workplace activism remained without sanctions, while the SSA could not reach frontline staff, and the RCN refrained from workplace activism completely.

6.3.2 Findings: Germany

Ver.di targeted the issue of staffing levels at both the national and the local level. National understaffing trends (as described in Chapter 1) were also reflected in figures from the Charité hospital in Berlin. Between 1990 and 2017, the national average length of stay of patients dropped from 16.7 to 8.9 days (OECD 2020). The Charité outperformed these numbers, with an average length of stay of only 5.9 days in 2015 (Der Tagesspiegel 2015). In addition, since 2006, the total number of employees at the Charité has decreased by 7 per cent, while the number of cases treated increased by 18 per cent and the case mix, which indicates the severity of the cases, by 23 per cent (IP33: 5, 14).

Trade unionists at the Charité complemented the national-level legislative campaign by organizing and mobilization, as well as networking with local civil society actors to achieve a collective agreement on safe staffing. Important pre-conditions for their activities were resources that were built up over years, but also deliberately developed during the campaign, and their effective use.

6.3.2.1 Resources and capabilities

The case of the struggle for staffing levels at the Charité has to be regarded in the light of a long employment relations history in which ver.di experienced a decline in institutional power at the hospital. However, ver.di trade unionists managed to generate strength from this situation, using it as an opportunity structure to change their strategy and compensate with building up organiza-tional power and developing a strong activist core. Local industrial relations collapsed from the mid-2000s onwards, when the Charité management decided to leave the employer's association ("Tarifgemeinschaft deutscher Länder", TdL) in 2006, which eliminated collective bargaining coverage by the TdL for the Charité employees. Following this, ver.di forced negotiations over pay by staging a two-week strike. In this way, ver.di managed to ward off a deterioration of pay rates and prevented a collective agreement on restructuring and cost savings (Sanierungstarifvertrag), in which workers usually approve wage constraints to give management room for restructuring the hospital. In 2011, after a successful strike, ver.di finally also managed to assure (re-)connection to the public sector collective bargaining agreement (TdL). This paved the path for a strike for safe staffing levels since a new strike concept was developed, facilitating strikes in the particularly sensitive hospital sector. In this concept, instead of guarantee-ing emergency staffing, the trade union announced the planned strike three to seven days beforehand and the responsibility to reduce bed capacities accord-ingly or to shut down entire wards lay with the hospital management (IP33: 7, 28; IP26: 12, 90, 92; IP37: 40).

The drop in institutional power and deterioration of employment relations at the Charité continued when ver.di started its campaign for safe staffing levels and revealed its rising organizational power. The Charité management rejected the legitimacy of regulating staffing levels within the framework of a collective bargaining agreement, as demanded by ver.di, with reference to entrepreneur-ial freedom (Art. 12 GG). Only after ver.di called for a warning strike in 2014 did management agree to negotiate at all. Due to the employer's reluctance to regulate staffing levels in a collective bargaining agreement, ver.di agreed to an arbitration settlement that mandated an increase in nursing staff by 80 full-time equivalents. However, this was not sufficient and was never properly imple-mented. Following the strike and arbitration settlement, the research services of the German Bundestag stated that the demand for staffing level regulations as part of health protection in collective bargaining agreements was legal, and the Berlin Labour Court confirmed this. The described conflicts were accompanied by warning strikes in 2006, 2011, and 2013. Ver.di then engaged in a second round of negotiations from 2013 onwards, which are the central subject of this case study (IP33: 10; Int. IP26: 20, 22, 37, 84, 102).

In short, the conflict about pay and first attempts to regulate staffing were important experiences for ver.di to learn, to improve their collective bargaining position, and to develop a strong activist core group. This source of associational power was then used and further developed as part of an organizing strategy in the struggle for staffing levels. In the same way, ver.di deliberately built up its source of societal power by founding the Charité alliance as part of a social movement unionism strategy. These processes will be presented in the next section dealing with ver.di's strategies.

Finally, trade unionists at the Charité benefited from additional support provided by ver.di at the national level and the national campaign The Pressure must be Released (Der Druck muss raus), as well as a general understaffing campaign that addressed deteriorating working conditions of nurses and lobbied for statutory staffing levels. Initially, these campaigns were to be complemented by negotiations of staffing levels in collective agreements in selected hospitals, and this is the setting within which the Berlin campaign emerged. However, the national trade union structures shifted the focus of the campaign to the demand for statutory staffing levels due to the enormous variety of collective agreements in public, private for-profit, and private not-for-profit hospitals. Nevertheless, ver.di trade unionists at the Charité were supported at the national level (IP33: 7; IP26: 14, 17, 20, 84; IP37: 32, 39, 85, 100).

6.3.2.2 Strategies

The national-level campaign that accompanied activities at the Charité focused on lobbying politicians for statutory staffing levels and smaller publicity actions at the hospital level, as well as the provision of expertise through surveys on staffing and working conditions, such as the Ver.di Night Shift Assessment (ver.di Nachtdienstcheck) and the Ver.di Personnel Assessment (ver.di Personalcheck) (IP37: 27, 34, 45, 50), which could also be used by the union at the Charité Berlin.

At the level of the Charité, ver.di showed good capabilities to actively develop their organizational and societal power resources. This allowed using a variety of different strategies, with a special focus on workplace and community organizing. As described in the previous section, ver.di developed the organizational prerequisites for an activist organization by engaging in the 2006 and 2011 strikes. It built up a core group of activists, developed a new strike concept, staged several strikes and also improved their strike position through the legal clarification of striking against understaffing as part of health protection of workers.

Thereafter, ver.di consolidated its associational power by mobilizing nurses to participate through the so-called emergency call (Notrufkonzept) and collective agreement consultant (Tarifberater) concepts. With these emergency calls, entire wards can give notice of a dangerous work overload. In contrast to similar concepts in the English and US American case studies, it needs to be stressed that these notices were not filed individually, but collectively, and linked to consequences if hospital management did not improve the situation; nurses could announce a work-to-rule after a specified period of time.

The second crucial concept for mobilizing and including the workforce in the struggle for staffing levels since 2013 has been the inclusive communication structure of the collective agreement consultants. It is worth noting that the function of collective agreement consultants could also be filled by non-members. Trade unionists, with the support of the Charité alliance (see below), went around the wards and convinced employees to participate in seminars. In these seminars, supported by the Charité alliance, activists explained the links between the hospital reimbursement system of the DRGs and the work intensification for employees. Some of these participants then took over the task of the collective agreement consultants, thus functioning as disseminators and communicating what happened at the negotiating table to their wards. In this way, activists came together for regular meetings and had the opportunity to give feedback on the current status of the negotiations, gradually building up an activist organization (IP33: 28, 60, 61; IP26: 93, 96; IP37: 41). Through the collective agreement consultants, ver. di introduced a deliberative element into collective bargaining, and thus showed another capability that helped to mobilize resources effectively – associational power in this case.

Ver.di further mobilized nurses by addressing their professional ethic that usually inhibits their willingness to strike. Ver.di effectively reframed this ethic and altered the local union's identity toward a more class-based orientation. They depicted nurses as empowered actors: nurses' professional ethic makes them prone to strike because they realize that working under prevailing working conditions does not allow them to provide good service to their patients. In this way, ver.di successfully mobilized nurses for strike action and also discovered their previously underrated workplace bargaining power. A relatively small number of nurses who were willing to go on strike had a strong effect due to already insufficient staffing. In the Charité, 300 striking nurses (out of 4,200 nurses) were sufficient to reduce the services to an ethically responsible minimum (IP33: 36). In the 2015 strike, more nursing staff were ready for work stoppages than was ethically and legally acceptable (IP27: 102).

Apart from the mobilization of its members, the development and the use of societal power was an important source of ver.di's strength. Ver.di Berlin showed a good network capability and deliberately increased its societal power by founding the Charité alliance "Berliners for More Personnel in the Hospital" (Berlinerinnen und Berliner für mehr Personal im Krankenhaus). Developing and using the resource of the Charité alliance was enabled through a wider framing of the conflict as a sociopolitical issue (IP33: 5, 7, 12, 14, 52, IP26: 20, 48, 94, IP37: 11, 15, 17, 75). Ver.di activists founded the Charité alliance in 2013 to increase support and publicity for their collective bargaining negotiations. Even though the number of alliance members declined over time, the alliance remained active and met regularly. It consisted of people from leftist and socialist independent political groups, of individuals that belonged to the doctors' associations VdÄÄ ("Verein demokratischer Ärztinnen und Ärzte", Association of Democratic Doctors) and Marburger Bund, to the leftist political party (Die Linke), activists from other hospitals, ver.di officials, Charité works councilors and activists, a patient organization, and interested individuals.

With support of the alliance, ver.di could mobilize other stakeholders besides the nursing staff, and communicate demands to the public more easily. Ver.di activists and trade unionists framed the understaffing issue as deliberate work intensification through an output-orientation initiated by the DRGs, staff reductions in the 1990s and cost pressures due to insufficient investments in infrastructure. Moreover, according to the activists, this broad social issue required the creation of "counter-norms" which redirect resources to the workforce. This issue framing was successful and disseminated by the Charité alliance to mobilize community members in addition to union members (IP33: 5, 7, 12, 14, 52, IP26: 20, 48, 94, IP37: 11, 15, 17, 75). Based on the support of the Charité alliance that became an established and well-known actor in Berlin, the conflict also received good coverage in the media. This was further helped by the publication of extensive information through different channels, such as press releases, press conferences, a webpage, as well as a Facebook account (IP27: 35, 84, 105). The local newspaper Der Tagesspiegel regularly published articles on the Charité and the issue of staffing levels. The strike in 2015 also received national media attention (IP33: 52).

Furthermore, the alliance developed its own political practice supporting safe staffing levels. Initially, the alliance was only a support alliance for the strikes over pay. Because the strike in 2013 was delayed several times and there was the collective agreement arbitration result that entailed a peace obligation until the end of 2014, the alliance developed its own political agenda. This led to initiating a petition that asked for the inclusion of quality regulations in the form of staffing levels in Berlin's state hospital plan (Landeskrankenhausplan). The alliance managed to politicize this otherwise rather non-political administrative act and achieved Berlin-wide media attention (IP33: 38, 39, 44, 48, 50, 60; IP26: 22, 51, 62, 66, 68, 70; IP27: 17, 19, 21, 23, 32, 35, 37, 43, 45, 46, 60–64, 77, 95, 107, 109). Nevertheless, the petition did not lead to binding staffing levels (Der Tagesspiegel 2016), and therefore was followed by an initiative for a referendum that started in early 2018. For the trade union activists, the alliance was a useful resource, for instance for practical support or expertise on innovative strategies (IP26: 48; IP27: 60).

Moreover, ver.di tried to use institutional power and lobbied ministers, health policy groups and workers' groups at the level of local Berlin politics, where the Social Democrats and Conservatives governed the Berlin Senate from 2011 until 2016. However, this strategy did not appear to be overly important or effective. Only the announcement of the strike gave the trade unionists greater leverage and finally led to a meeting with the Berlin Senator for Health, Mario Czaja (CDU), in which ver.di activists together with the Charité alliance presented their demands for safe staffing levels and sufficient hospital funding in the state hospital plan. These demands, however, were not fulfilled (IP33: 9, 46; IP26: 62–64, 76, 80; IP27: 77), and, as mentioned above, this was followed up by a referendum initiative in 2018. Furthermore, at the workplace level, ver.di utilized its institutional power and pursued a more cooperative strategy by contributing its expertise in the development of detailed patient-to-staff ratios for different functional divisions, to be laid down in the collective agreement (IP26: 36, 38).

In these ways, ver.di Berlin was able to create an activist organization, build up and tap into workplace, community, and media resources, as well as mobilize nurses through an empowerment identity and sociopolitical framing.

6.3.2.3 Outcome

The above-described strategies resulted in several significant gains. On the statutory level, the topic of safe staffing levels was put on the political agenda. Ver.di was invited to a public hearing on the issue in the German national parliament in March 2015. After the hearing, the German national parliament set up an expert commission to investigate the relation between nurse workloads and care quality, and developed a procedure to determine and introduce minimum staffing levels for "care-sensitive" medical departments (Bundesministerium für Gesundheit 2017). Moreover, due to the activities at the Charité, the legal situation has been clarified and a new opportunity to strike for health protection on a national scale established.

Additionally, and arguably most importantly, at the level of collective regulation, ver.di Berlin successfully concluded a collective agreement at the Charité that obliged the employer to increase staff numbers at the end of April 2016 (ver. di 2016). This agreement concerned all hospital workers and mainly consists of patient-to-staff ratios. It also introduced procedures in cases of heavy workload, especially for areas in which no patient-to-staff ratios could be defined, as well as a regulation concerning the maximum share of untrained workers allowed on the wards. Moreover, a newly instated health committee with its own budget was to monitor compliance with the collective agreement and to decide on measures to be taken in case of work overload procedures (ver.di Charité Tarifkommission 2015). However, in autumn 2017, the Charité activists regarded it as necessary to go on strike and renegotiate details on the implementation of the collective agreement on staffing levels (Heine 2017).

Last, but not least, the activities at the Charité have spilled over to other hospitals. The municipal hospitals of Berlin launched the Standing Together (ZusammenStehen) campaign at the end of 2015, in which they demanded safe staffing levels as well (ver.di 2015a, b) (IP27: 110–116; IP30: 66, IP24: 53, 65). Until the end of 2020, ver.di concluded agreements on safe staffing levels in nearly 20 large German hospitals, most of them university clinics.

6.3.3 Findings: New York State

Similarly to the German and English cases, NYSNA was confronted with understaffing trends at the state level, as well as the national level. New York State rolled out a managed care program for Medicaid recipients in 1997 with the Partnership Program 1115 Waiver, and in 1998, managed care was extended to long-term care services (Center for Medicare & Medicaid Services (CMS) n.d.). State-wide hospital occupancy rates dropped from 82.8 per cent in 1983 to 65.3 per cent in 2004 (Berger 2006). These cost pressures are compounded especially for hospitals that have a high proportion of Medicaid, Medicare and uninsured patients, which tend to be smaller community hospitals as well as the New York City Health and Hospitals Corporation, a public hospital system set up in 1969 (IP48). They tend to be in competition with not-for-profit academic medical centres based in Manhattan that serve a larger proportion of patients with commercial insurance and provide more lucrative services due to their status as academic medical centres (ibid.).

These increased cost pressures have led to the closure of 70 hospitals between 1983 and the early 2000s (Berger 2006), as well as another 19 hospitals between 2000 and 2013 in New York State (Caruso 2013). Moreover, hospitals have responded to these pressures by downsizing inpatient services, outsourcing ancillary services such as environmental health services, and merging into larger hospital-based health systems, leading to increased consolidation in the market. Another measure has been to privatize hospitals under public ownership (see, e.g., Frost 2016 for the case of the Long Island College Hospital, LICH).

For the safety net and public hospitals that remain open, the hospital closures have led to a large increase in the volume of patients being admitted to Emergency Departments and inpatient wards. This is because the Medicaid and uninsured patients previously seen at small community hospitals are now receiving their care at these safety net and public hospitals (IP49). As part of the New York Campaign for Patient Safety, NYSNA documented 18,557 Protests of Assignment, in which nurses provide formal notice to an employer that their assigned workload is unsafe. Around 85 per cent (15,808) of those Protests of Assignment occurred in or close to New York City, where most hospital closures have also occurred.

6.3.3.1 Resources and capabilities

When analyzing NYSNA's resources and capabilities, as in the case of ver.di Berlin, the younger history of activism should be considered. The prevention of hospital closures and previous multi-employer bargaining were important experiences that helped increasing institutional and associational power. One of NYSNA's most important responses to the cost pressures prevailing in the sector has been to build up its associational power and transform its organizational structure toward an activist organization This occurred in the context of a dynamic opportunity structure. First, Andrew Cuomo was elected New York State Governor in 2010, taking over a deficit of $10bn in the State budget. Cuomo set up a team of experts to redesign New York State's Medicaid program, the most expensive in the USA. The Medicaid Redesign Team put a global spending cap on the Medicaid budget, established a program targeting high-risk

Medicaid recipients and initiated a reform of Medicaid's payment mechanism (Medicaid Redesign Team 2011), all of which intensified the cost pressures and market consolidation mentioned above. In addition, Bill de Blasio, the first Democratic New York City Mayor since 1993, was elected in 2013 with strong support from NYSNA (see further below).

In the midst of these political and healthcare changes, activist reformers and members transformed NYSNA's organizational structure, and thus also its own identity from a professional, market-oriented association into a mobilizing, more class- and society-oriented trade union (Brenner 2015). NYSNA was founded in 1901 and up until 2011, largely acted as a professional association, providing its members with information and educational opportunities, and lobbying State Assembly members (Brenner 2012). Moreover, nurse managers had dominated the board of directors, limiting the executive direction that it could provide in union matters (due to labor law restrictions). In response, reformers campaigned in favor of militancy and member mobilization, and won nine out of thirteen board seats in elections in 2011 (Brenner 2011). An important reason for their election victory was that members felt the previous, management-dominated leadership was out of touch with what bedside nurses cared about. Their concerns predominantly included dealing with too many patients and the associated problem of unregulated staffing levels (IP53), the trend of downsizing inpatient wards and the associated job losses for RNs (IP54), as well as a lack of protection afforded by strong workplace representation and a union contract in public sector hospitals, especially after the 2007/2008 financial crisis had been stabilized (IP55). In May 2012, NYSNA members voted for bylaw changes to establish a trade union model focused on bargaining, mobilization and community campaigning that became effective in October 2012 (IP50). The final pivotal organizational restructuring came at the end of 2012, when the new NYSNA board hired Jill Furillo as NYSNA's new Executive Director. Before joining NYSNA, Furillo was the Government Relations Director for the California Nurses Association (National Nurses United 2012) and successfully led the campaign for staffing regulations in California. Moreover, she had previously been the Executive Vice President of 1199SEIU's RN Division, meaning she had developed ties with many important stakeholders in New York City and knew the regional context well (IP54).

NYSNA furthered its class-oriented identity not only through organizational changes but also through a specific framing. To mobilize its union members NYSNA has framed healthcare issues as class-based sociopolitical problems, and called on an empowerment identity that conceptualized worker interests as a function of community interests. Achieving resonance with such class-based empowerment identities is important because traditional nursing identities posit that engaging in militant practices constitutes a neglect of patients. To avoid this issue, NYSNA organizers first made sure that actions at the workplace level, such as petitioning management or groups of members calling on management to change their practices, preceded militant public actions, so that militancy appeared as a legitimate last resort. Second, organizers also made it clear that diverting attention away from patients to the public for a few days is preferable to regularly providing patients with poor care due to understaffing (IP54). Especially the 2011 reformers emphasized that achieving gains is only possible through the empowerment of nurses in a trade union that shows its strength in numbers (Brenner 2011). An empowerment identity rejects passive sacrifice, for example in faith-based nursing (Reich 2012), instead evoking images of (military) power: "We became an army determined to see quality care delivered to all our patients" (NYSNA 2016f) and of political and social change: "We advocate for the patients and we are considered the agents of change" (IP49). NYSNA emphasized that nursing is about protecting families and entire communities (NYSNA 2016a), so that adequate staffing ratios and working conditions become a matter of protecting community needs rather than a matter of self-interest (IP50). As evidence, citations of academic research showing how having more RNs improves care usually accompany this frame (NYSNA 2015a). NYSNA embedded this empowerment identity in a framing of problems related to healthcare, such as inadequate access or medical errors as a result of social inequalities. The common slogan "Patients before Profits" expresses the class-based nature of this social justice frame. NYSNA has criticized hospital closures, downsizing services and market consolidation as inimical to satisfying patient needs (NYSNA 2016f). Part of this frame is also NYSNA's critique of racial disparities and poor healthcare access for underserved communities (NYSNA 2016c).

In addition to its increase in associational power and a shift in union identity, NYSNA could also draw on some institutional power, the multiemployer bargaining, that became well-established over the previous years. New York State's hospital sector has traditionally been more coordinated due to a strong Department of Health regulating the supply of services through Certificate of Need regulations, but also through the trade union 1199SEIU organizing healthcare workers since around 1959 and engaging in multiemployer bargaining since 1969 (IP51). 1199SEIU has 200,000 members in New York State and it won a collective bargaining agreement through multiemployer bargaining with the League of Voluntary Hospitals and Homes of New York in July 2014 (1199SEIU 2014). This agreement applies to around 46 healthcare organizations and their establishments, and it includes reviews of RN staffing guidelines. Though there is some overlap between the two unions, 1199SEIU's membership consists to a large degree of unlicensed workers in private sector organizations, while NYSNA has around 12,000 of its 37,000 union members in public sector organizations and predominantly organizes licensed nursing professionals ('RNs').

Furthermore, during the course of the looming hospital closures of LICH and of Interfaith Medical Center, NYSNA made important learning experiences and built up its power resources (NYSNA 2016f). On their own initiative and with little leadership support, NYSNA activists had fought a campaign against service downsizing at LICH in 2008. In 2013, by contrast, NYSNA prioritized the campaign. As the then city councillor for Brooklyn, Bill de Blasio also supported this campaign (Semente n.d.), NYSNA drew on his support in public demonstrations, but also in the context of a NYSNA-supported lawsuit in 2013 at the Supreme Court against the LICH closure. Already at this point, NYSNA established a network of actors supporting their cause. To raise awareness and put pressure on city officials, NYSNA partnered with churches, school and community groups, as well as healthcare advocacy groups for protests, town hall meetings, leafletting and putting up flyers in local businesses (IP50). Moreover, the organizer assigned to the campaigns started to mobilize LICH's non-RN staff that was unionized under 1199SEIU. Additionally, Jill Furillo employed her ties to motivate 1199SEIU officials to join the campaign. The two unions subsequently worked closely together (1199SEIU 2013, NYSNA 2016e), and, in 2014, they commissioned the Community Strategy Lab for the study "Caring for Today, Planning for Tomorrow" that made recommendations on restructuring Interfaith Medical Center based on a community needs assessment. Governor Cuomo subsequently took on some of the restructuring proposals and funded a three-year pilot project to keep the centre open (IP57).

In addition to community organizing, NYSNA has built up its associational power and workplace presence through a network of nurse representatives who support a group of elected RN leaders (delegates and bargaining unit executive committee officers), and whose work is coordinated by regional area directors. This structure has relied heavily on member initiatives and participation (IP58). Moreover, while the previous management-driven board had deprioritized new organizing, the new board designated organizing as a priority in 2013. This consisted of identifying suitable nurse leaders, developing their skills in an organizing committee, supporting them in having one-to-one conversations with other workers to convince them of voting for the union, and using home visits only when necessary due to their high investment (IP54).

Associational power, but also institutional power was further build through multiemployer bargaining. After drawing on Bill de Blasio's support during the LICH campaign and supporting him in his election, NYSNA signed a collective bargaining agreement with his new administration in June 2014 for their public sector members (IP50). NYSNA's decision to attempt multiemployer bargaining in 2015 was a pivotal moment in driving the focus on workplace organizing. The decision to coordinate bargaining negotiations across multiple employers built on 1199SEIU's long history of multi-employer bargaining in New York State. Multiemployer bargaining was also a way for NYSNA to leverage its workplace power because it unified members in multiple locations (IP54). NYSNA first negotiated multiemployer bargaining with four big hospital-based health systems and subsequently extended the negotiations to thirteen other health systems. To get management to agree to multiemployer bargaining, NYSNA opened up negotiations to all members, but had to agree that the negotiations would be in a hotel, away from any hospital campus. Moreover, Jill Furillo had convinced a negotiator who had worked for 1199SEIU to temporarily come out of retirement and act as NYSNA's lead negotiator (IP56). Because management could not agree on a proposal by mid-April 2015, NYSNA coordinated a day of picketing across the four health systems and held a press conference to publicize management's lack of willingness to settle (NYSNA 2015b). In response to management's continuing unwillingness, NYSNA balloted its members and received a 90 per cent strike authorization (ibid.), which prompted a settlement in mid-June 2015. Similar to 1199SEIU's 2014 agreement, NYSNA's agreement established Professional Practice Committees with the purpose of reviewing "standards of nursing practice" (Memorandum of Agreement 2015), monitoring "staffing guidelines for each unit" (ibid.) and receiving reports about float pools. However, the agreement also permitted NYSNA to engage in informational picketing about staffing issues, to put public pressure on management, thereby institutionalizing their right to more militant tactics. The 2015 multi-employer campaign was also significant because NYSNA subsequently repeated the use of coordinated picketing to renew contracts. At Nathan Littauer Hospital in Upstate New York, NYSNA responded to a management lock-out with a four-day strike in early January 2016. However, this was ineffective, and only coordinated picketing with strike authorizations in two other hospitals of the same health system prompted management to agree to a settlement (IP54). In mid-2016 NYSNA also successfully coordinated picketing across three Catholic hospitals in Long Island (NYSNA 2016b).

6.3.3.2 Strategies

Once the organizational prerequisites for class-based activist strategies had been established, NYSNA moved to deploying their new resources by re-orienting their practices toward more on-the-ground organizing and a stronger focus on the public realm (IP56). Accessing and mobilizing regional resources as well as the successful framing of an empowerment identity were necessary for successfully implementing activist strategies.

An important component of organizing was a focus on community organizing that drew on politicians, the media, and other civil society groups. In December 2012, NYSNA launched its campaign to prevent the closures as practiced in the aforementioned hospital closure campaigns.

In addition to on-the-ground organizing, NYSNA has started "advocating at a public level for patients" (IP58) to achieve statutory regulation of staffing. NYSNA supported Black Lives Matter through a white coat march in March 2014 and it worked together with Healthcare Now and the Physicians for a National Health Program on single payer healthcare and the prevention of hospital closures (IP49). This collaboration fostered NYSNA's network. The union in turn could also rely on support for their demands from the according groups. To amplify its messages and put pressure on public officials, NYSNA has organized TV journalists to cover protests, rallies and informational pickets. NYSNA has also contributed to newspaper articles (Robbins 2015) and used advertisements and press conferences to put pressure on management during bargaining in pay and professional practice committees to ensure safe staffing, and on public officials for its legislative campaigns. NYSNA has used its ties to numerous State Assembly Members for support of its legislative campaigns (IP49) as well as its ties to city councillors and public officials at public events (NYSNA 2016f). NYSNA has also published a lengthy contribution to consultations in preparation of a Medicaid waiver program as well as providing clinical and workforce input at most of the waiver's regional implementation committees (IP60).

Along with its bylaw changes in mid-2012, NYSNA re-launched a campaign aimed at legislative changes that would enable the New York State Department of Health to require minimum patient-to-nurse staffing ratios. While there have been similar attempts since the early 1990s, the fact that NYSNA could not mobilize many members to pressure lawmakers meant these campaigns remained ineffective (IP56). The 2012 campaign also consisted of lobbying New York State Assembly members to back the Safe Staffing for Quality Care Act. However, this time NYSNA was able to use the momentum from its multi-employer bargaining pickets to mobilize 1,000 members to visit the State Assembly on the 21st of April 2015 to lobby for the legislation (New York State Assembly 2016). NYSNA has also started to collect data on staffing ratios in which NYSNA members report the staffing ratios they encounter on their shifts via text message on a daily basis to provide quantitative evidence of the extent of understaffing (IP52).

Finally, NYSNA launched the New York Campaign for Patient Safety in February 2016 that is a coalition made up of trade unions and community advocacy groups in favor of safe staffing (NYSNA 2016a). The campaign has so far focused on producing videos about the need for safe staffing and reports summarizing the research on the effects of staffing regulations.

The class-based orientation was not only reflected in the framing, but also in videos, press releases, legislative memos, and other documents NYSNA published and which reflected the stance that access to healthcare was a fundamental right that should not depend on ability to pay (NYSNA 2016d). In mid-2016, NYSNA formed the Social Justice Committee to work more systematically on social justice issues, with its initial work focused on conceptualizing gun violence as a health issue (IP58).

6.3.3.3 Outcome

NYSNA pursued its main strategic goal of preventing understaffing by focusing more on community and workplace organizing to prevent hospital closures and build up workplace power to enforce collective bargaining agreement provisions (including staffing guidelines). Moreover, NYSNA has focused more on the public realm through public protests, involvement in broader healthcare activism, and its legislative campaign for mandated staffing ratios.

These strategies required an organizational transformation led by reformers who responded to member concerns that the previous leadership had not met. Once these organizational prerequisites were met, NYSNA built up its resource base through workplace representation networks and new organizing, but also by engaging public officials, the media, and other civil society organizations to build up pressure for its campaigns. Additionally, adopting some of the tactics of and working closely with the incumbent healthcare union 1199SEIU led to a multiemployer contract that provided further institutional resources (e.g., the right to picket and professional practice committees). Furthermore, to overcome barriers from anti-militant nursing identities and to meet member concerns, NYSNA had to employ empowerment and social justice frames.

The strategies described have led to important gains. NYSNA's multiemployer contract provided wage increases, added around 1,000 new full-time equivalent RN positions, and secured or extended float pools. In addition to establishing professional practice committees, the agreement also included provisions to secure RN employment, meaning that nurses working in units to be downsized must be reassigned to other units in the hospital (Memorandum of Agreement 2015).

Gains through NYSNA's legislative campaign have been more limited. The NYSNA-sponsored Safe Staffing Bill passed the Assembly on the 14th of June 2016 and moved onto the Senate stage (New York State Assembly 2016). However, this also constituted an improvement, considering that the bill had not moved forward in the last two decades.

6.4 Comparisons

Fitting the most-different systems approach, this section will very briefly compare the cases from England and Germany and, in more detail due to their strong parallels, the German and US American cases.

In all cases under study, unions were confronted with work intensification and aimed at easing workloads and improving patient safety by bringing the issue to public attention, working in alliances with other stakeholders. In England, this was complemented only by weak demands for mandatory staffing levels and workplace activities. In Germany and the US, unions pursued a complementary workplace strategy, strongly involved nurses, and showed a more self-confident, confrontational attitude, following a society- and class-oriented identity. Both unions used a wider sociopolitical framing of the issue that helped mobilize nurses despite their strong professional ethos.

Most striking in comparison to the cases from Germany and the US, is that in the English case neither the unions nor the SSA pursued a rigorous mobilization of nurses in the workplace. This might be due to the fact that unions and other stakeholders in the sector did not succeed in developing a joint demand. The blurred objective of improving staffing was probably more difficult to organize and mobilize upon. In addition, especially UNISON showed a strong market-oriented framing and cooperative attitude that did not allow challenging policymakers and employers, and that was also less suited to encouraging nurses to become more active and militant. Even though unions and stakeholders in England recognized the political opportunity following the care scandals, they fell short on on-the-ground organizing. In the case of UNISON, this can be explained with scarce resources, but also with a lacking belief in the potential of mobilizing nurses.

In contrast to initiatives in England, unions in Berlin and New York State focused on strong grassroots and membership participation, and practiced union democracy. Their strategy included also non-organized workers in their communication structure and other activities. Their society- and class-oriented identities allowed for a broader framing and concerted action with allies to exploit the existing societal power to push for their interests. None of the unions shied away from confrontation with either employers or policymakers.

Eventually, both NYSNA and ver.di Berlin were successful with their strategy of collective regulation in the pursuit of staffing levels. Moreover, the same factors have enabled them to do so. In order to mobilize staff and members, both unions recently transformed their organizations into activist organizations. Both unions recognized and used specific opportunity structures: while in the New York case, this transformation relied on 1199SEIU's long history of multiemployer bargaining as well as reform and bylaw changes, in Berlin the transformation occurred due to management leaving the employers' association, a move to which ver.di Berlin responded with strikes. However, both paths have led to activist organizational structures that were subsequently employed in collective bargaining and public legislative campaigns.

Additionally, both unions enjoyed good access to the media, healthcare activists, community groups and local politicians, enabling them to mobilize external stakeholders to their advantage. One difference is that ver.di Berlin seems to have had less access to politicians than NYSNA. However, overall both unions have been successful at mobilizing external stakeholders. Additionally, the more beneficial access to employers that German codetermination usually affords unions did not provide ver.di Berlin with leverage, because the Charité management refused to negotiate over staffing at the workplace level. Only when the Parliamentary research services had declared staffing to be a legitimate topic of bargaining and the Berlin Labour Court ruled the legality of strikes about staffing levels in the hospital sector, did the Charité management engaged in treating the topic of staffing levels in collective bargaining.

Another important factor concerns the framing of issues as broader sociopolitical issues rather than just workplace issues. Though NYSNA also incorporated a social justice frame that addressed racial inequalities in healthcare, and ver.di Berlin had focused mostly on socioeconomic dimensions, both unions have been able to speak to members' and patients' concerns over poor quality of care due to deteriorating working conditions. By tying worker and patient interests together, both unions have overcome the conservative view that unions are purely self-interested.

Moreover, by calling on a nurse identity that emphasizes patient advocacy, agency, and empowerment, both unions have also overcome an issue that professionalism runs into: the inability to mobilize members for actions due to their identification as self-sacrificing, passive carers. While ver.di Berlin has built up the confidence to engage in political actions gradually through successful strikes, NYSNA tended to use rallies, picketing and community organizing to evoke an empowerment identity. In its 2015 round of collective bargaining NYSNA members also voted in favor of strike action, but did not need to follow through as hospital managers agreed to negotiate a multi-employer agreement.

6.5 Conclusion

In this chapter, the institutional determinants of trade union strategy was examined, drawing on evidence from nurses' unions in England, Germany, and the USA. The findings showed that trade unions could leverage local institutional legacies by transforming their organizations into activist organizations, leveraging resources such as the access to local politicians, the media, healthcare activist networks, and community members, framing issues as sociopolitical problems to mobilize community members, and by calling on an empowerment identity as a source of member mobilization. In these ways, trade unions can successfully mobilize stakeholders internally and externally to create coalitions against management practices that endanger safe working conditions and patient safety such as understaffing in the healthcare sector. In England, it was mostly the market-identity and a cooperative approach without an institutional power basis, as well as the inability to arrive at unified demands with other unions and stakeholders, that prevented the effective use of resources. Finally, the campaigns failed to include and mobilize members, let alone organize non-unionized nurses.

The research design is robust and generalizable in so far as the findings refer to nurse union strategies because the same factors driving successful union strategies were identified in two very different national systems of industrial relations and healthcare. However, the research design focused predominantly on nurse unions at the regional level and may thus not be applicable to national-level union actions. Moreover, some findings, such as the condition of overcoming a subordinating and self-sacrificing professional identity, may be specific to the healthcare sector. However, ver.di's organizing strategies have already spread to other hospitals, and NYSNA's collective bargaining successes have increased the coordinated character of the New York State healthcare system. Furthermore, though calling on an empowered nurse identity may be specific to healthcare, the need to overcome the view that unions are only self-serving and pit workers against consumers is a long-standing issue (Simons 1944) and a barrier to unionization. Aligning the interests of workers and consumers/patients, as nurse unions have done, is a key finding of this chapter that applies to union campaigns more generally.

The findings of this chapter imply that there is some space for trade unions to exert agency. Unions can actively build up resources in their community, such as through coalitions with activists, they can change their organizational structures, and they can use appropriate frames and call on appropriate identities to mobilize members. Both ver.di's establishment of a workplace-based communication network along with its use of strike tactics and NYSNA's rapid transformation of its organizational structure into a social movement union model show that such agency can be considerable and can result in fundamental changes in a short space of time. However, apart from member and staff resistance to such changes (Voss and Sherman 2000), lacking political allies in the community may limit the amount of agency trade unions can exert (Gindin 2016).

The problem of understaffing for nurses is one which will likely continue across all healthcare systems of the advanced economies because of financial problems associated with aging, higher acuity patients, and cost containment. Because staffing levels are easily communicated and understood, and the experience of dangerous staffing levels erodes nurses' main aim of high-quality patient care, staffing levels may form an adequate basis for promoting international standards and the enforcement of such standards.

Note

1. However, in its 100-year history as professional organization and 40-year history as a trade union, the RCN, to date, never went on strike (National Health Executive 2017).

References

1199SEIU. 2013. Members of 1199 and NYSNA Arrested at SUNY Offices Delivering Save LICH Petition. http://www.1199seiu.org/members_of_1199_and_nysna_arrested_at_suny_offices_delivering_save_lich_petitions#sthash.oZ6u34eD.dpbs.

1199SEIU. 2014. Members of 1199 and NYSNA Arrested at SUNY Offices Delivering Save LICH Petition. http://www.1199seiu.org/members_of_1199_and_nysna_arrested_at_suny_offices_delivering_save_lich_petitions#sthash.oZ6u34eD.dpbs.

Aiken, Linda H., Douglas M. Sloane, Luk Bruyneel, Koen Van den Heede, and Walter Sermeus. 2013. Nurses' Reports of Working Conditions and Hospital Quality of Care in 12 Countries in Europe. *International Journal of Nursing Studies* no. 50 (2):143–153.

Aiken, Linda H., Jeannie P. Cimiotti, Douglas M. Sloane, Herbert L. Smith, Linda Flynn, and Donna F. Neff. 2011. Effects of Nurse Staffing and Nurse Education on Patient Deaths in Hospitals with Different Nurse Work Environments. *Medical Care* no. 49 (12):1047–1053.

Aiken, Linda, Douglas M Sloane, Luk Bruyneel, Koen Van den Heede, Peter Griffiths, Reinhard Busse, Marianna Diomidous, Juha Kinnunen, Maria Kózka, Emmanuel Lesaffre, Matthew D McHugh, M T Moreno-Casbas, Anne Marie Rafferty, Rene Schwendimann, P Anne Scott, Carol Tishelman, Theo van Achterberg, and Walter Sermeus. 2014. Nurse Staffing and Education and Hospital Mortality in Nine European Countries: A Retrospective Observational Study. *Lancet* no. 383:1824–1830.

Ash, Michael, Jean A. Seago, and Joanne Spetz. 2014. What Do Health Care Unions Do?: A Response to Manthous. *Medical Care* no. 52 (5):393–397.

Auffenberg, Jennie, and Nick Krachler. 2017. Arbeitsverdichtung im Krankenhaussektor: Erfolgreiche gewerkschaftliche Strategien zur Personalbemessung. *WSI-Mitteilungen* no. 4/2017:269–277.

Ausserhofer, Dietmar, Britta Zander, Reinhard Busse, Maria Schubert, Sabina De Geest, Anne Marie Rafferty, Jane Ball, Anne Scott, Juha Kinnunen, Maud Heinen, Ingeborg Strømseng Sjetne, Teresa Moreno-Casbas, Maria Kózka, Rikard Lindqvist, Marianna Diomidous, Luk Bruyneel, Walter Sermeus, Linda H. Aiken, and René Schwendimann. 2013. Prevalence, Patterns and Predictors of Nursing Care Left Undone in European Hospitals: Results from the Multicountry Cross-Sectional RN4CAST Study. *BMJ Quality & Safety* 23 (2). http://qualitysafety.bmj.com/content/23/2/126.

Berger, Stephen. 2006. A Plan to Stabilize and Strengthen New York's Health Care System. http://www.nyhealthcarecommission.org/final_report.htm.

Brenner, Mark. 2011. Reformers Sweep Election in New York Nurses Union. *Labor Notes.* http://labornotes.org/2011/09/reformers-sweep-election-new-york-nurses-union.

Brenner, Mark. 2012. New York Nurses Take Back Their Union, Push for Safe Staffing. *Labor Notes.* http://labornotes.org/2012/05/new-york-nurses-take-back-their-union-push-safe-staffing.

Brenner, Mark. 2015. New York Hospitals on Notice. *Labor Notes.* http://labornotes.org/2015/05/new-york-hospitals-notice.

Briskin, Linda. 2012. Resistance, Mobilization and Militancy: Nurses on Strike. *Nursing Inquiry* no. 19 (4):285–296.

Bundesministerium für Gesundheit. 2017. Schlussfolgerungen aus den Beratungen der Expertinnen- und Expertenkommission "Pflegepersonal im Krankenhaus". Berlin. https://www.bundesgesundheitsministerium.de/fileadmin/Dateien/3_Downloads/P/Pflegekommisison/170307_Abschlusspapier_Pflegekommission.pdf.

Caruso, David B. 2013. NYC's Neighborhood Hospitals Closing as Financial Pressures Mount, Part of Larger Trend. *Associated Press, August* 6.

Center for Medicare & Medicaid Services (CMS). n.d. Managed Care in New York. https://www.medicaid.gov/medicaid-chip-program-information/by-topics/delivery-systems/managed-care/downloads/new-york-mcp.pdf.

Clark, Darlene A., and Paul F. Clark. 2006. Union Strategies for Improving Patient Care: The Key to Nurse Unionism. *Labor Studies Journal* no. 31 (1):51–70.

Clark, Paul. F., and Darlene A. Clark. 2003. Challenges Facing Nurses' Associations and Unions: A Global Perspective. *International Labour Review* no. 142 (1):29–47.

Clark, Paul. F, Darlene A. Clark, David V. Day, and Dennis G. Shea. 2001. Healthcare Reform and the Workplace Experience of Nurses: Implications for Patient Care and Union Organizing. *Industrial and Labor Relations Review* no. 55 (133): 133–148.

Cook, Andrew, Martin Gaynor, Melvin Stephens Jr., and Lowell Taylor. 2012. The Effect of a Hospital Nurse Staffing Mandate on Patient Health Outcomes: Evidence from California's Minimum Staffing Regulation. *Journal of Health Economics* no. 31 (2):340–348.

Dube, Arindrajit, Ethan Kaplan, and Owen Thompson. 2016. Nurse Unions and Patient Outcomes. *Industrial & Labor Relations Review* no. 69 (4):803–833.

Francis, Robert. 2013. Report of the Mid Staffordshire NHS Foundation Trust Public Inquiry: Executive Summary. London: The Stationery Office.

Frost, Mary. 2016. Brooklyn Judge Finalizes Sale of Long Island College Hospital. *Brooklyn Daily Eagle, January 30.*

Gindin, Sam. 2016. Beyond Social Movement Unionism. *Jacobin.* https://www.jacobinmag.com/2016/08/beyond-social-movement-unionism/.

Gordon, Suzanne. 2009. Institutional Obstacles to Rn Unionization: How 'Vote No' Thinking Is Deeply Embedded in the Nursing Profession. *Working USA* no. 12 (2):279–297.

Griffiths, Peter, Chiara Dall'Ora, Michael Simon, Jane Ball, Rikard Lindqvist, Anne-Marie Rafferty, Lisette Schoonhoven, Carol Tishelman, and Linda H. Aiken. 2014. Nurses' Shift Length and Overtime Working in 12 European Countries: The Association With Perceived Quality of Care and Patient Safety. *Medical Care* no. 52 (11):975–981.

Gruber, Jonathan, and Samuel A. Kleiner. 2012. Do Strikes Kill? Evidence from New York State. *American Economic Journal: Economic Policy* no. 4 (1):127–157.

Heine, Hannes. 2017. Pflegestreik wirkt – Klinik verzeichnet Umsatzeinbußen. *Der Tagesspiegel, 21 September, 2017.* http://www.tagesspiegel.de/berlin/charite-in-berlin-pflegestreik-wirkt-klinik-verzeichnet-umsatzeinbussen/20361528.html.

Jennings, Karen, and Glenda Western. 1997. A Right to Strike? *Nursing Ethics* no. 4 (4):277–282.

Kane, Robert. L., Tatyana A. Shamliyan, Christine Mueller, Sue Duval, and Timothy J. Wilt. 2007. The Association of Registered Nurse Staffing Levels and Patient Outcomes: Systematic Review and Meta-Analysis. *Medical Care* no. 45 (12):1195–1204.

Keogh, Bruce. 2013. Review into the Quality of Care and Treatment Provided by 14 Hospital Trusts in England: Overview Report. London: NHS.

Lafer, Gordon. 2005. Hospital Speedups and the Fiction of a Nursing Shortage. *Labor Studies Journal* no. 30 (1):27–46.

Medicaid Redesign Team. 2011. A Plan to Transform the Empire State's Medicaid Program. Better Care, Better Health, Lower Costs. https://www.health.ny.gov/health_care/medicaid/redesign/docs/mrtfinalreport.pdf.

Memorandum of Agreement. 2015. Memorandum of Agreement By and Between the NYC Hospital Alliance and NYSNA. June 19.

Moody, Kim. 2014. Competition and Conflict: Union Growth in the US Hospital Industry. *Economic and Industrial Democracy* no. 35 (1):5–25.

National Health Executive. 2017. RCN Threatens First Strike in 100-Year History Over 1% Pay Cap, May 15. http://www.nationalhealthexecutive.com/Health-Care-News/Page-110/rcn-threatens-first-strike-in-100-year-history-over-1-pay-cap.

National Nurses United. 2012. Jill Furillo, RN, Joins New York State Nurses Association as Executive Director. *Press Release, November 29.* http://www.nationalnursesunited.org/press/entry/jill-furillo-rn-joins-new-york-state-nurses-association-as-executive-direct/.

New York State Assembly. 2016. Assembly Passes Safe Staffing for Quality Care Act. 2016, June 15. *NY Assembly Press Release.* http://nyassembly.gov/Press/20160615/.

NYSNA. 2015a. Memo of Support. AN ACT to Amend the Public Health Law, in Relation to Enacting the "Safe Staffing for Quality Care Act." https://www.nysna.org/sites/default/files/attach/1317/2015/01/A1548S782SafeStaffing.pdf.

NYSNA. 2015b. New York Nurse. https://www.nysna.org/sites/default/files/attach/1522/2015/08/NYNurse_JulyAug.pdf.

NYSNA. 2016a. Legislative Briefing on Safe Staffing Packs Room. http://www.nysna.org/legislative-briefing-safe-staffing-packs-room#.V4lfCLh97IU.

NYSNA. 2016b. Nurse Unity on LI. https://www.nysna.org/nurse-unity-li#.WLYZ-TsrI2x.

NYSNA. 2016c. Nurses Reflect on Black History Month. http://www.nysna.org/nysna-nurses-reflect-black-history-month#.V4lbxLh97IU.

NYSNA. 2016d. NYSNA Nurses Campaign for Safe Staffing at Black and Puerto Rican Caucus. http://www.nysna.org/nysna-nurses-campaign-safe-staffing-black-and-puerto-rican-caucus#.V4lagbh97IU.

NYSNA. 2016e. Two Unions. One Heart. http://www.nysna.org/two-unions-one-heart#.V4lbjLh97IU.

NYSNA. 2016f. Video: '2015 Year in Review'. http://www.nysna.org/video-%E2%80%982015-year-review%E2%80%99#.V8THtpgrLIW.

OECD. 2020. Health care utilisation. https://stats.oecd.org/Index.aspx?DataSetCode=HEALTH_PROC.

Rafferty, Anne Marie, Sean P. Clarke, James Coles, Jane Ball, Philip James, Martin McKee, and Linda H. Aiken. 2007. Outcomes of Variation in Hospital Nurse Staffing in English Hospitals: Cross-Sectional Analysis of Survey Data and Discharge Records. *International Journal of Nursing Studies* no. 44:175–182.

RCN. 2014. An Uncertain Future: The UK Nursing Labour Market Review 2014. https://www2.rcn.org.uk/__data/assets/pdf_file/0005/597713/004_740.pdf.

Reich, Adam. 2012. *With God on Our Side. The Struggle for Workers' Rights in a Catholic Hospital*. Ithaca/London: ILR Press.

Robbins, Alexandra. 2015. We Need More Nurses. *New York Times*, May 28. http://www.nytimes.com/2015/05/28/opinion/we-need-more-nurses.html.

Safe Staffing Alliance. 2017. The Alliance. http://www.safestaffing.org.uk/the-alliance/.

Schreyögg, Jonas. 2016. Expertise zur Ermittlung des Zusammenhangs zwischen Pflegeverhältniszahlen und pflegesensitiven Ergebnisparametern in Deutschland im Auftrag des Bundesministeriums für Gesundheit (BMG). https://www.bundesgesundheitsministerium.de/fileadmin/Dateien/5_Publikationen/Pflege/Berichte/Gutachten_Schreyoegg_Pflegesensitive_Fachabteilungen.pdf.

Seago, Jean. A., and Michael Ash. 2002. Registered Nurse Unions and Patient Outcomes. *The Journal of Nursing Administration* no. 32 (3):143–151.

Semente, Julie. n.d. How We Saved Our Hospital. http://www.nysna.org/how-we-saved-our-hospital#.V4lWybh97IU.

Simons, Henry C. 1944. Some Reflections on Syndicalism. *Journal of Political Economy* no. 52 (1):1–25.

Tagesspiegel, Der. 2015. Immer weniger Pflegekräfte für immer mehr Patienten. http://www.tagesspiegel.de/politik/notstand-in-den-krankenhaeusern-immer-weniger-pflegekraefte-fuer-immer-mehr-patienten/11955050.html.

Tagesspiegel, Der. 2016. Neuer Berliner Krankenhausplan: Mehr Geld, Betten und Personal für die Gesundheit. *Der Tagesspiegel*. http://www.tagesspiegel.de/berlin/neuer-berliner-krankenhausplan-mehr-geld-betten-und-personal-fuer-die-gesundheit/12923962.html.

ver.di. 2015a. Bei Vivantes geht's los. *ver.di Infodienst Krankenhäuser*, 21–22.

ver.di. 2015b. Neues von Vivantes. *ver.di Infodienst Krankenhäuser*, 28–29.

ver.di. 2016. Urabstimmung bei der Charité endet mit eindeutigem Ergebnis: ver.di stimmt Tarifvertrag Gesundheitsschutz und Mindestbesetzung zu http://bb.verdi.de/presse/pressemitteilungen/++co++4ac3ee60-0d3a-11e6-8c40-525400438ccf.

ver.di Charité Tarifkommission. 2015. Tarifvertrag Gesundheitsschutz zu Ende verhandelt: Alle ver.di Mitglieder zur Urabstimmung aufgerufen. http://www.mehr-krankenhauspersonal.de/1795.

Voss, Kim, and Rachel Sherman. 2000. Breaking the Iron Law of Oligarchy: Union Revitalization in the American Labor Movement. *American Journal of Sociology* no. 106 (2):303–349.

7 Trade unionism in times of marketization

7.1 Introduction

This chapter aims to draw conclusions from the synthesis of the four empirical chapters presented in this book. It intends to summarize the determinants of trade union strategies and to formulate prospects for trade unionism in the marketized health sector. In the first section, the main findings of the empirical chapters will be presented in a generalized way. The implications of these findings for the theoretical approach will be reviewed, and a refined theoretical model, suitable for studying trade union strategies in times of health sector marketization, will be presented in the following section. To conclude, the contribution of the book, its shortcomings, as well as gaps that need to be filled by further research will be discussed in the last section.

7.2 Main empirical findings

This book aimed to identify the determinants of (successful) trade union strategies in conflicts arising from different forms of marketization in the hospital sector. To this end, 19 case studies were presented in four empirical chapters, drawing on a total of 137 interviews and approximately 800 documents. The empirical chapters were dedicated to the three main forms of privatization (corporatization, outsourcing, and material privatization), in addition to trade unions' attempts to contain their effect of work intensification through mandatory staffing levels. Unexpectedly, unions made comparable strategic choices despite their two most-different settings in terms of welfare and employment relations systems – England and the USA as representatives of the liberal market economy type and Germany as a representative of the coordinated market economy type. This hints at the mediating effect of marketization trends on employment relations institutions and highlights the importance of the recognition of sector-specific political opportunities, as well as local unions' resources and capabilities.

The first empirical chapter (Chapter 3) examined two cases of formal privatization of large-scale hospitals in the capital cities of Germany and England in the early-2000s. In both cases, the issue was not politicized, and trade unions opted for a partnership approach to prevent negative effects for employees. However, the outcomes of the two corporatization processes were very different. Ver.di, using a proactive partnership approach and suggesting alternatives while credibly threatening to resort to legal confrontation, achieved far-reaching agreements on codetermination rights, job security, working conditions, and pay. This was possible through an agreement with the employer to commission a consultancy in the restructuring process that ensured the inclusion of the trade union and the employees. Through the consultancy, ver.di activists and works council received training in the business side of hospital management and, in this way, could increase its salient knowledge. The inclusion of employees and ver.di members in the process, foreseen and moderated by the consultancy, introduced deliberative elements which also strengthened the union. Ver.di recognized corporatization as an opportunity structure through which it could achieve its own objectives, i.e. the merger of the municipal hospitals to avoid competition among them, and to increase their sustainability.

The institutional framework guaranteeing systematic inclusion and code-termination of the union in the formal privatization process was lacking in the English case. For this reason, in line with the comparative employment relations theory, the English unions would not have been expected to choose a partnership strategy. Nevertheless, following a strong market-oriented union identity, UNISON strongly relied on its weak institutional power and chose a partnership approach while leaving other resources, such as strong associational power that would have allowed for complementary strategies, unused. However, when analyzing the English case of corporatization, the national setting needs to be considered as well. The introduction of the Agenda for Change (AfC) coincided with the corporatization. The AfC secured wages of workers and further toned down the politicization of corporatization. This revealed the potentially weakening effects of national regulations for local trade unionism. The generally low political salience of formal privatization in England might further explain why UNISON did not exhaust its power resources. However, formal privatization has a low level of politicization in Germany, too. It could also be argued that UNISON, in contrast to ver.di, failed to recognize the corporatization process as an opportunity to further workers' interests.

These case studies highlighted the importance of matching resources to strategies, as well as formalization of the partnership and a complementary strategy – two of the preconditions brought forward by Fichter and Greer (2004). Furthermore, the case studies showed how the union's identity (Hyman 2001) determines its strategic repertoire. UNISON's market-oriented identity determined the strategic choice of partnership, despite lacking institutional power resources. Last, but not least, the unions perceived corporatization in different ways. Ver.di recognized it as an opportunity (Gamson and Meyer 1996) to influence hospital reorganization in the workers' interest.

The second empirical chapter (Chapter 4) presented evidence from two case studies of support services outsourcing in two large hospitals in Germany and

England from 2015 to 2017. Again, the main strategy of both unions was partnership. In these case studies, the partnership strategy was combined with organizing efforts to retain outsourced members and organize new workers. Also in the outsourcing process, the partnership strategy was pursued regardless of adverse framework conditions. UNISON's market-oriented identity again restricted its repertoire of contention. This time, however, UNISON initially also deployed some social movement strategy elements. These attempts were ceased after the outsourcing had taken place. Ver.di, in turn, increased its activity post-outsourcing and used the local opportunity structure to join forces with activists fighting for the insourcing of the subsidiary of another big hospital in Berlin, the Charité.

With additional support from its structures at the national level, UNISON managed to retain its outsourced membership and establish union structures in the new company. However, since a formalization of the partnership was missing, trade union representatives soon complained about little influence in the service company. In the same way, UNISON observed that their agreement based on the recently diluted national Transfer of Undertakings (Protection of Employment) Regulations (TUPE) was circumvented by the private provider. Thus, working conditions and pay deteriorated, and workers became increasingly dissatisfied with their new employer. Protests intensified as a response to unacceptable hygiene standards in the hospital, which were caused by poor results of the cleaning services. These protests were led by a national grassroots campaign group. As a result, the hospital insourced the services to improve hygiene standards only two years later.

Ver.di, in turn, partly managed to resist outsourcing, as it negotiated dynamic validity of their previous collective agreement for outsourced workers and started negotiating another collective agreement for new workers. The union actively included workers in these processes and succeeded at mobilizing its membership for protests and strikes. Moreover, the union did not cease its activity after collective bargaining, but even increased its efforts. Contrary to what would have been expected considering typically high institutional power, ver.di ended its partnership approach. The union used the local opportunity structure and teamed up with their colleagues at the Charité in a campaign to align new workers' terms and conditions with those of the transferred workers and pursued the insourcing of all services. Their strategic approach was transformed into social movement unionism post-outsourcing, drawing on societal power and exploiting the increasing public attention for union struggles at hospitals in Berlin. However, after two years of fighting, the union had not reached its goals. The case study, nevertheless, showed the local leeway for unions and the possibility of increasing salience of functional privatization and its revaluating effect on societal power resources as pointed out by Ganz (2009). Furthermore, in England, the fight for the insourcing of the service was not considered by the union. Instead, this was fought for by a grassroots campaign group. The German case is also an example of how framing can create political opportunities (Gamson and Meyer 1996). Framing insourcing as a possible option and an enduring attitude allowed the union to mobilize both the workers and the public.

The third empirical chapter (Chapter 5) studied all large-scale privatizations of hospitals in Germany since 2004 and, correspondingly, all the cases of outsourcing of medical services above a £60m value in England from 2014 to 2016. This chapter also showed that marketization specificities of the sector must not be neglected. The funding of healthcare and the healthcare market structures can both unfold effects that might superimpose other macroinstitutional structures. Subsequently, theories referring to these structures might not adequately describe healthcare sector employment relations in practice. Considering these sector-specific structures and marketization processes can help reveal political opportunities and allow the use of certain capabilities that mobilize resources, for instance by framing privatization of hospitals as a threat to the national health system to mobilize public support, as happened in England. Moreover, English anti-privatization campaigners benefited from a fundamental reform that attracted public attention and from inexperienced purchasers and politicians in the newly established Clinical Commissioning Groups, who were vulnerable to public protest. Ver.di, in turn, was struggling with a very indirect link between the introduction of the diagnosis-related groups (DRGs) and the incentives for privatization they created. Healthcare funding as such was rarely criticized prominently by the unions. The DRG reimbursement system and its privatization incentives gradually took effect in the sector, and ver.di only started responding when the privatization trend was fully underway. Consequently, ver.di was unsuccessful in preventing the privatization in the majority of cases, even though the union succeeded at mobilizing public support and demanding concessions from the hospital owners with regards to the transfer of workers. A more anticipatory, proactive and preventive strategy appeared more suitable in the cases of hospital privatization. The late case of the Dresden municipal hospitals, which were about to be formally privatized, can serve as an example. Ver.di had learned from earlier cases that corporatization was usually followed – sooner or later – by the hospital's sell-off. Furthermore, ver.di also had learned that referenda are not effective if they are not binding. Therefore, ver.di Dresden first rendered referenda binding and then had the citizens decide about both the formal and the anticipated material privatization. In addition, ver.di suggested alternatives for the further development, a merger of the hospitals, to ensure their sustainability.

The case studies in England also demonstrated that grassroots campaign groups, a force that was less present in the German cases, can play a powerful role in preventing privatization. Unions in England joined grassroots campaigns in those places where they existed before the trade union anti-privatization activities had begun. This is a variation of social movement unionism, in which unions usually lead an alliance of union supporters. The grassroots groups had their own repertoires of contention, which enriched the unions' strategies. Furthermore, in some cases, grassroots campaign groups were even successful without much union involvement, and thus regardless of the union density in the corresponding hospitals. These grassroots campaigns provide a chance for unions to frustrate privatization attempts despite low unionization rates. The results of this chapter indicate the importance of wider public protest and the potential for the tactics of new social movements. However, the effectiveness of this strategy revealed its limits when in 2016 a large medical services contract in England was commissioned to Virgin Care by a Conservative majority in the local council. This might be due to falling salience of the topic after the 2015 general election or due to an increased confidence of the Conservatives after their general election victory. It could also reflect a learning process on the part of purchasers and commissioners.

The case studies of the third empirical chapter have drawn attention to sector-specific marketization processes that may overlap with national employment relations institutions, similar to what has been demonstrated by scholars of liberalization theory (Katz and Darbishire 2000; Bordogna 2008; Baccaro and Howell 2011;). These processes may create political opportunities that can be used by anti-privatization campaigners. The capability for learning (Lévesque and Murray 2010) proved to be important for all actors involved in privatization cases. The topic of hospital and medical services privatization appeared to be of high public interest, a resource that could be exploited not only by unions, but as the English case has shown, also by other civil society groups. The character of sector-specific marketization policies affected their salience, supporting what has been described by Culpepper (2010) and Ganz (2009). The capability for framing privatization as a threat and the capability for networking (Frege and Kelly 2003; Lévesque and Murray 2010) allowed unions to mobilize societal power and to work in coalitions.

The fourth empirical chapter (Chapter 6) presented three cases of campaigns for staffing levels, to ease work intensification as an effect of corporatization, outsourcing, privatization, and other cost pressures in the sector. The comparison of campaigns for staffing levels in Germany and England that took place between 2013 and 2016 in large metropolitan hospitals was complemented with a third case from New York State (2012 to 2016) due to its surprising and striking parallels to the German case. The English case turned out to be unsuccessful, while in the German and US American cases, ver.di and New York State Nurses Association (NYSNA) achieved collective agreements on mandated staffing levels. In these cases, unions were – consciously or subconsciously – deploying their capabilities considerably more systematically, and thus were more effective at mobilizing and developing their resources in comparison to the previous cases.

Ver.di, as well as NYSNA, successfully brought their organizational power to its full effect by means of deliberative organizational structures and encouragement of workplace-level activism. In this way, the unions developed communication networks to disseminate information and receive feedback on decisions to be taken in the collective negotiations and mobilized members to notify their employers of work overloads. NYSNA, a nursing union with a history of professionalism, even changed its identity from market- to class-oriented, and thus it developed into an activist organization open to militancy. Ver.di and NYSNA also both deployed a framing of the understaffing issue in wider social justice terms. This mobilized important societal resources, allowed for cooperation in a network of allies and created additional media attention.

Last, but not least, especially ver.di used a broad spectrum of strategies, although they differed in the extent to which they were employed, this nevertheless proves that a combination of strategies is possible. Ver.di contributed expertise in the development of the patient-to-staff-ratios, which can be regarded as part of a partnership approach, while also organizing and mobilizing members. At the same time, ver.di also cooperated with allies from civil society and worked on increasing the public pressure. Thus, thanks to a good basis of resources that had been developed throughout previous conflicts and the struggle for staffing levels, ver.di was able to use various strategies and deploy them flexibly.

The English case, in turn, again revealed the importance of a match between resources and strategies. It also again confirmed the high preconditions that need to be fulfilled for a partnership to be successful. Despite a lack of institutional power, UNISON decided for a partnership approach and only targeted the issue of understaffing and encouraged employees to file complaints in cases where hospital employers agreed to it. UNISON failed to combine this approach with a more proactive and complementary strategy, and it did not place it in a broader social agenda. Furthermore, UNISON's campaign was not coordinated with the Safe Staffing Alliance – potentially suitable to activate societal power – it participated in.

The case studies of the struggles for staffing levels in Germany and New York State were very similar in strategic choices and outcomes. This again hints to the importance of local-level factors, as pointed out by Locke (1992). These local-level factors seemed to be more decisive than national employment relations regimes due to common marketization trends and corresponding pressures on the workforce. The cases also pointed to the importance of a union's identity (Hyman 2001), its changeability, and determining influence on strategic choices. The unions' adoption of a more militant identity also supports recent findings on trade unionism in health and social care services that refute the argument of a low organizing potential in female-dominated professions and among female workers (Artus et al. 2017). In addition, both unions benefitted from practising a democratic and deliberative culture of trade unionism, as described by Lévesque and Murray (2010) and Ganz (2000).

To summarize, in all case studies trade unions made strategic choices that were both surprising and untypical from a traditional comparative industrial relations theory perspective. In the cases of union responses to corporatization and outsourcing of support services (Chapters 3 and 4), the English union unexpectedly opted for a partnership approach that appeared unfit given their systematic lack of institutional power. This choice can be explained with a low political salience of these forms of marketization, as well as a specific market-oriented identity and the consequent framing of the problem as a practical constraint that was not to be questioned. This specific identity and framing were inadequate to mobilize their strong associational and societal power resources, namely high union density and strong public support for public healthcare provision. Their relative defeat can be attributed to a mismatch of the strategic choice and actual power resources. In the campaigns against privatization and for mandatory staffing levels (Chapters 5 and 6), the German union unexpectedly adopted, in most of the cases, a social movement strategy that is typical for unions in liberal market economies. A specific framing of the problem in terms of social justice and a society-oriented identity was suitable for building up and mobilizing both associational and societal power, i.e. to mobilizing both employees and other stakeholders. Due to the specific structure of the health sector, which includes both private and public ownership of hospitals, and given the strong and institutionalized role of politicians in privatization processes, the German union was usually not successful with this strategy with respect to this form of marketization. Nonetheless, it has to be noted that the German union successfully mobilized the workers and the public, and it usually obtained major concessions from employers that secured employees their pay and working conditions. Furthermore, in more recent cases, ver.di seemed to have learned to anticipate privatization threats and managed to take measures to prevent them. In the English case, privatization was prevented when the unions worked in collaboration with grassroots initiatives, used the sector-specific opportunity structure of the newly established Clinical Commissioning Groups and a lack of experience of commissioners and purchasers, framed the issue in terms of social justice, and followed a suitable social movement unionism approach. In the most recent case of the fight for mandatory staffing levels, the German union was successful with its social movement strategy. This might be due to increased salience of the issue in an advanced marketization environment, the proactive nature of the endeavor or due to the implementation of the strategy in combination with extensive membership inclusion.

Strong parallels in the cases studied hint at a need for a distinct classification of the health sector, independent from the usual welfare state and employment relations typologies. Due to its profound marketization, the German health sector experiences cost pressures and creates problems comparable to those in health sectors in liberal market economies. The more marketization advances, the more promising trade union strategies typical for liberal market economy settings seem to be.

In addition, in contrast to comparative industrial relations theory, considerable local-level variation could be found in the strategic choices, especially in the different German cases. This additionally supports the thesis that national institutions do not fully determine local-level employment relations, but the importance of local-level resources and capabilities instead. Furthermore, unions deployed a combination of strategies in their outsourcing and understaffing campaigns. Strategic flexibility seemed to be important for success and their simultaneous deployment (Chapter 6) was more effective than using them successively (Chapter 4).

Instead of deducing from welfare state typologies and focusing on the determining character of national-level institutions, this book tries to explain unions' strategic choices with sector-specific opportunity structures stemming from marketization processes and with local-level resources and capabilities. In a more general sense, it aims to shift the focus from national-level structures to local-level agency of unions. Welfare state typologies cannot explain the choice of partnership strategies in England despite an absence of suitable institutional resources. The specific trade union identity appears more suitable to explain this phenomenon. In the same way, German unions would be expected to be influence-oriented and focus on their traditionally strong institutional resources. However, the more marketization intensifies, the more relevant the power resource of societal power became. Marketization processes appear to have a transformative impact on employment relations, independent of changes in formal institutions, similar to what has been described by Katz and Darbishire (2000) and Baccaro and Howell (2011). With increasing intensity, marketization conflicts seem to generate similar pressures and outcomes, which might hint at a convergent trajectory of trade unionism in the healthcare sector across different countries and the potential of sharing best union practices internationally.

The next section will refer back to the theoretical approach of this book and will suggest a refined theoretical model based on the empirical evidence.

7.3 Theoretical implications: A model of political opportunities and local-level determinants of trade unions' strategic choices

After having summarized and compared the main findings from the empirical chapters, the theoretical implications will be assessed in this section.

The empirical analysis has shown considerable local-level variation in strategies and unexpected strategic choices that call into question theories focusing on national structures. These need to be extended by local agency factors. To account for this agency, it is worth emphasizing the role of marketization-induced political opportunities and their recognition, the use of associational and societal power, and finally the mobilization of these power resources through the capabilities of framing and identity, organizational practice and leadership, as well as networking.

To analyze trade union strategic choices in conflicts about marketization and its effects, I therefore suggest an extension, reorganization, and refinement of the Frege and Kelly (2003) model to reconcile the theories presented in Chapter 2 with the empirical findings on trade union strategies of this book. Strategy in this model is understood as the means to achieve a purpose. Resources are deployed to attain an objective. Capabilities improve the effective and efficient use of these resources. Strategy is further understood as a choice and not deterministically. Therefore, strategies can also be deliberately changed. Nevertheless, I acknowledge that critical choices are often made unconsciously and incrementally through processes of debate and compromise.

The model is based on the assumption that strategic choice derives from an interaction of local and sector-specific factors, as opposed to the traditional

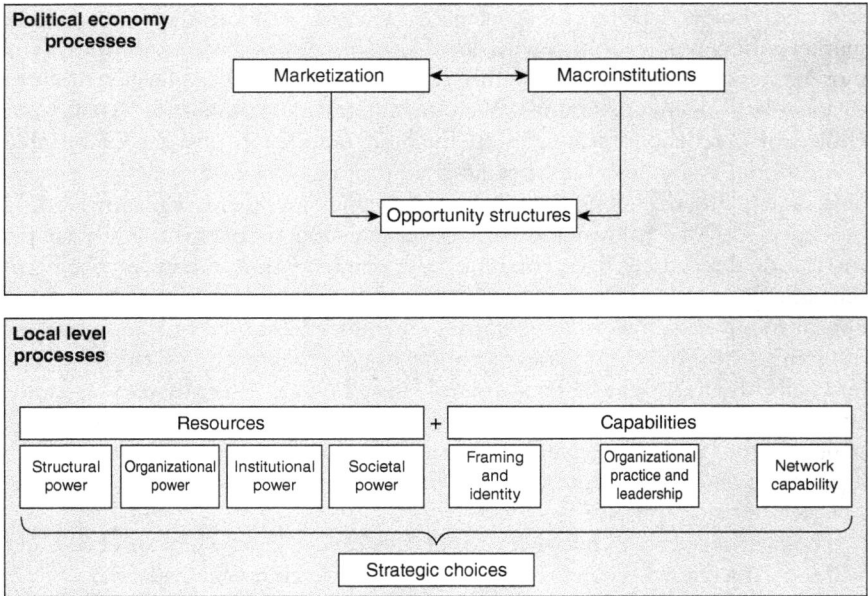

Figure 7.1 A model of political opportunities and local-level determinants of trade unions' strategic choices in times of marketization.

industrial relations research that stresses macroinstitutional determinants. It considers marketization as creating an opportunity structure, or, in other words, creating comparable pressures to prevent a deterioration of pay, working conditions, and quality of care, that allows trade unions to use new strategies, independent of the institutional setting they are acting in. Trade union strategies then depend on local-level factors, such as the local union's endowment with power resources, the union's identity, its framing of the problem under consideration, organizational practice and leadership, as well as the union's networking capabilities (see Figure 7.1).

Marketization, as a profound political economy process, changes the environment in which trade unions operate. This can alter the effectiveness of traditional trade union strategies that formerly matched the macroinstitutional setting. Therefore, when analyzing the choice of trade union strategies and their effectiveness, it is worth taking marketization trends into account and thinking beyond traditional macroinstitutional determinants. Furthermore, these marketization-induced changes can create new opportunities. Marketization processes can put unions in a defensive position; they can, however, also be used as a chance for revitalization. Unions can participate in restructuring processes, devise new strategies, and mobilize workers and the public around marketization issues. This potential for revitalization can be used by trade unions if they recognize the opportunity and possess, or alternatively manage to build up, the necessary capacities and power resources to change their traditional strategic behavior and deploy new strategies.

Applied to the health sector, marketization processes create opportunity structures in two ways. First, marketization needs to be implemented, and has effects, at the local level. Trade unions can intervene in the restructuring processes that marketization creates at the hospital level, for instance changes in legal form, outsourcing or material privatizations (see Chapters 3, 4, and 5). Second, marketization increases competition and creates strong cost pressures that translate into work intensification (see Chapter 6). This will in turn affect the quality of care. The health sector is of high public interest, which means that the salience of political issues in this sector is also high. Both work intensification and declining care quality can create psychological strain and a need for action among employees as well as the public. This can result in exit, but it can also increase workers' voice. This latter potential can be used to increase trade union power resources – associational and societal power in particular. They can be mobilized through a suitable framing of the problem in terms of social justice and a corresponding society- or class-oriented trade union identity, a deliberative organizational practice and diverse leadership team, as well as cooperation with allies from civil society. Given the increasingly marketized nature of the health sector, typical strategies used in liberal market economy settings, such as social movement unionism and organizing, seem most adequate considering the available power resources.

In the next section, the theoretical findings will be used to formulate possible implications, keeping in mind the empirical evidence.

7.4 Practical relevance and implications for hospital sector unions

This section will now assess the practical relevance of the findings and draw conclusions from the proposed theoretical model as well as the empirical evidence for future actions by trade unions in the hospital sector. The section will begin with the political economy processes and then place a special focus on the organizational-level processes that also deserved most attention in the empirical analysis. The section will conclude with an attempt to further classify and relate resources, capabilities, and strategies to one another.

7.4.1 Political economy processes: Plasticity and sector-specificity of employment relations regimes

As has been shown, the healthcare sector in both England and Germany experienced profound marketization and privatization. These processes provoked competition and cost pressures that manifested to a similar extent in their liberal and coordinated market economies, respectively, contrary to what theories focusing on a stable macroinstitutional setting would suggest. Drawing on system-level differences, i.e. the union's institutional embeddedness, as suggested by the Varieties of Capitalism framework, Baccaro, Hamann, and Turner (2003) expected differing responses of German and British unions to competitive pressures. German unions were expected to be disincentivized from "mobiliz[ing] their membership [...] build[ing] coalitions with other groups, or giv[ing] support to grass-roots initiatives" (p. 121) due to "adequate institutional supports" (p. 119). British unions, in turn, were expected to compensate for a weak institutional position by building coalitions and mobilizing members. As described above, German and British unions in the health sector responded in similar ways to different forms of marketization and privatization. In the cases studied, ver.di and, unexpectedly, also UNISON, chose a partnership strategy in less politically salient forms of privatization, i.e. corporatization and outsourcing (Chapters 3 and 4). Ver.di pursued complementary strategies that involved mobilization of members. In the more politically salient forms of privatization and its effects, i.e. hospital and medical services sell-offs and understaffing, both unions focused on membership mobilization and building coalitions (Chapters 5 and 6). To summarize, there is no clear pattern that would systematically distinguish trade unions' responses in the hospital sectors of the two countries studied. The choice of strategies seems to rely more on the form of privatization and local-level factors that will be discussed later.

The health sectors under investigation do not only stand out from welfare state theories because of the strong role of public sector health services in Britain's allegedly liberal regime (Bambra 2005), but also because they do not adequately capture the dynamics of marketization and privatization processes that can bring about radical changes in short periods of time (Hauptmeier 2012, 740).

As found for the metal and telecommunications industries (Hassel 1999; Doellgast and Greer 2007), in the health sector, marketization and privatization can lead to profound changes as well. When hospital services are outsourced or hospitals privatized, unions experience a change in their power resources. They lose parts of their institutional power if services or hospitals are run by a new provider, and thus they are confronted with a new employer. Organizational power is weakened because of a workforce dualization. Collective bargaining becomes more fragmented. Since "there is a gap between institutional rules and their enactment" (Streeck and Thelen 2005, 50) that gives actors "some leeway in deciding" (Behrens, Hamann, and Hurd 2004, 24), new institutional rules or new institutions can provide new opportunities for trade unions, as for example in the case of the Clinical Commissioning Groups in Britain.

Furthermore, the trade unions studied are active in a sector that has a specific workforce structure, with a high share of part-time workers, female workers, and a special professional ethos, all of which need to be considered. Especially the professional ethos seems to be important and needs to be addressed in a specific way. It needs to be reinterpreted toward a more militant trade union identity and social justice framing, that combines demands for better working conditions with improvements in care quality, uniting interests of workers, patients, and the public, as has been shown in Chapter 6.

To sum up, the specificity of the healthcare sector and its dynamics must be followed closely and macroeconomic structures cannot be regarded as stable. This means that trade unions need to be attentive to changes in healthcare regulation, funding and provision, as well as to the possible opportunities they might yield, even though these developments appear as a threat demanding a defensive reaction at first glance. The studies presented in this book have shown that change can provide an opportunity and can be used to the benefit of unions' interest.

Even though the book places a special focus on the local level, it must be noted that marketization and its adverse effects originate from national-level policies and predominating neoliberal convictions. It is self-evident that the unions' leverage is greater if they are powerful enough to nationally and change profit- or austerity-oriented regulations toward the actual needs of patients, workers, and the public. Most prominently, as has been shown in Chapter 1, the abolishment of DRG system and replacement by a full cost coverage system would substantially alter the workings of the healthcare system. As main driver for marketization, privatization, work intensification, and declining care quality, the replacement of the DRG system would disincentivize the depicted marketization trends that work to the detriment of patients and workers and most probably reverse them. To give just one example, private providers would simply not be able to generate profits in the hospital sector in a full cost coverage system and thus be discouraged from economic activities in this sector.

As long as the trade union movement does not succeed altering the underlying problematic structures of the hospital sector's grievances, local-level struggles can mitigate marketization and partly avert its adverse effects. In this way, the collective agreements on staffing levels impede hospital managers from cost savings through reductions in personnel and in the case of private providers diminish the scope of profit making. At the same time, trade unions gain experience in organizing workers and raise awareness of the public. This can help addressing the underlying causes and increasing the pressure also at the national level at a later point in time.

7.4.2 Recognizing political opportunities

If unions are attentive to changes in the structures of the political economy and the possible opportunities they might provide for action, for their organization as unions, and to shape processes, then they have a chance to extend their influence on both, the national and local level. Times of change appear to be a good opportunity to suggest alternatives. A self-confident, anticipatory, and proactive union identity and behaviour seem to be of most benefit, as several case studies of this book have shown. Recognizing political opportunities requires salient knowledge (Ganz 2000) or a "capability to act" (p. 106), using the words of Nachtwey and Wolf (2013). Gamson and Meyer (1996) explored this idea further and argued that political opportunities can be created by an optimistic or even "unrealistic" framing in the sense of a self-fulfilling prophecy. The union's attitude toward a problem or a conflict as well as how they frame it appear important, and the targeted use of reframing seems worth considering.

The potential of the union's influence will then still depend on their resources and their capabilities to use them. The case studies on corporatization showed that whether a change is perceived as an opportunity and used as one depends very much on the trade union's identity.

7.4.3 Organizational-level processes: The mismatch between resources, capabilities, and strategic choices

Several case studies, especially in England, have brought up the problem of a mismatch between resources, capabilities, and strategic choices. Furthermore, resources were rather regarded as more static than dynamic. A closer look at the capabilities reveals their potential for the development and mobilization of these resources.

Therefore, an analysis and strategic build-up of resources using such capabilities seems to be useful. Furthermore, trade unions that could build on a broad basis of various resources and that possessed the capabilities to mobilize them were most successful. This granted them a high flexibility in their strategy choices that fit the appropriate situations and allowed for a simultaneous use of strategies that created particularly high pressure. The German corporatization case study has shown that a combination of partnership and more confrontational strategies can be expedient. The same holds for the US American and German case studies on understaffing, in which unions successfully concluded their agreements using a combination of organizing and social movement unionism, but also elements of partnership and lobbying.

Especially in times of changing environments, for example in times of marketization, capabilities are important for adapting to new conditions (Ganz 2000, Lévesque and Murray 2010). Therefore, an analysis of the resources should be combined with an analysis of capabilities. Capabilities are rarely discussed explicitly in the literature, but seem to be worth investigating further since they can help building and using power resources. Furthermore, capabilities can even compensate for a lack of material resources (Ganz 2000, 1041).

A strong belief in agency (Gamson and Meyer 1996) and the use of motivational framing (Benford and Snow 2000, 615 ff.; Kuypers 2009) appeared to be important for mobilizing the members, i.e. mobilizing the unions' associational power. This was most obvious in the German and US American cases of understaffing conflicts. Both unions showed a strong belief in agency. In the case of NYSNA, this was expressed in the development from a professional into an activist organization. Ver.di Berlin decided to fight for the first collective agreement on staffing levels despite scepticism of its legal feasibility. In the same way, the union pushed the boundaries for strike action in the health sector. Both unions further counted on nurses' willingness to strike despite their inhibiting professional ethos (Chadwick and Thompson 2000). They motivated nurses to strike by reinterpreting the professional ethos in a militant way (Wolf 2015). As such, nurses were compelled to strike in the patients' interest, so that the issue became politicized (Briskin 2012) and rationales for action were clearly laid out. The wider social justice frame that the unions used in these understaffing conflicts, but also in the cases of hospital and medical services privatization, enabled the use of new repertoires of action (Tarrow 2011) and facilitated building and using their societal power, i.e. networking with other stakeholders and using the social movement unionism strategy.

Union identities influence the way unions perceive changes as opportunities and threats (Hunt, Benford, and Snow 1994), and the strategies they choose (Hyman 2001). The English cases have shown how UNISON's business identity kept the union from bringing their resources to its full potential and using the whole spectrum of strategies and flexibly deploying them. Ver.di, in turn, often showed a more versatile identity that allowed for a flexible use of strategies, or at least for resorting to more confrontational measures when cooperative measures had no effect. A pure market-orientation of the union therefore seems to be less promising than a society- or class-orientation. Only the latter two orientations allow for a wider sociopolitical framing, mobilization of other stakeholders and, ultimately, the use of a variety of strategies and new repertoires of action. It might be worthwhile for the unions to reflect on their identity. Most remarkably, NYSNA has shown that an organization can change its identity over short periods of time if they use their democratic structures and replace leadership functions accordingly.

The capability of a diverse leadership was something only briefly discussed in this book due to little variation. Most interviewees were insiders, and thus did not extend the unions' repertoires of contention (Ganz 2000, 1014–1016). This might be worth considering and developing as well.

Deliberation and membership participation in decisions can give unions access to salient information, diverse points of view and ways of doing things, as well as provide an opportunity to learn. It can facilitate strategic innovation and can mobilize members, as well as strengthen their identification with the union (Ganz 2000, 1014 ff.). Deliberative procedures are particularly important in times of change since they are likely to provoke dissatisfaction and a desire to voice concerns (Hirschman 1970). The deliberative elements in the German outsourcing and understaffing cases helped motivating workers for action and increased their commitment in the conflict. There was no evidence that membership participation prolonged communication processes or undermined efficiency, as noted by Voss (2010, 377 f.).

Trade unions in the cases studied also learned from the past, for example when ver.di anticipated that formal privatization would entail material privatization and ensured that their referendum was legally binding before carrying it out. However, there was little evidence in the cases studied of a deliberate diffusion of new ideas for organizational practices, procedures, policies and programs, innovations to enhance resources, processes for membership engagement, use of new technologies, or new methods of recruitment as suggested by Lévesque and Murray (2010, 344 f.). Creating opportunities for the exchange and diffusion of best practices, also internationally, might help unions' building and using their resources most effectively, not only in anti-marketization campaigns.

Networking and collaboration with other civil society organizations can extend unions' financial and human resources, help connect to new groups of workers, complement their expertise, increase legitimacy of their demands, and facilitate mobilization of popular support (Frege, Heery, and Turner 2004, 139–141). In the cases studied, unions were not most likely to enter coalitions when associational and structural power were weak or in decline, as found by Frege, Heery, and Turner (2004, 145–149), but rather when their conflict was of public interest and sufficiently salient as in the anti-privatization and understaffing campaigns. However, it could be confirmed that a class or society orientation foster coalition building, as posited by Hyman (2001) and Turner and Hurd (2001). Potential partners generally seemed to be available as a precondition for coalition building, as pointed out by Gindin (2016) and Locke (1992). The local-level political parties were available as potential partners, as well as nongovernment organizations, such as patient organizations, leftist activist groups, or churches. Networking was clearly of crucial importance in the anti-privatization campaigns in England and Germany, and the understaffing conflicts in Germany and the USA. Since it can be a valuable asset, unions might want to foster their networking capability by winning activists and leaders with experience in other social movements, as suggested by Frege, Heery, and Turner (2004, 145–149).

A summary of the interaction of capabilities and resources, i.e. which capabilities appear to be helpful to build up and mobilize respective resources, is presented below (see Table 7.1).

Finally, differing strategies necessitate different resources and capabilities. Therefore, resources and capabilities should match strategic choices, or they should be built deliberately to provide an adequate basis for the strategy in order to be successful. Ideally, unions should have a broad basis of resources and should not neglect one resource in favor of another, possess the capabilities to activate each resource, and have a wide repertoire of contention they can choose from. In an increasingly economically liberal environment, unions used to cooperative strategies might be advised to extend their repertoire of contention, to be able

Table 7.1 Capabilities for mobilizing and fostering resources

	Structural power	Organizational power	Institutional power	Societal power
Framing		X		X
Identity	X	X	X	X
Organizational practice		X		
Leadership		X	X	X
Network capability				X

Source: Own presentation.

Table 7.2 Resource preconditions for different strategies

	Structural power	Organizational power	Institutional power	Societal power
Social partnership	Medium	Medium to high	High at workplace level	Medium
Organizing	Medium	High	Low	Low
Social movement unionism	Low	High	Low	High
Lobbying	Low	Medium	High at political level	High

Source: Own presentation.

to resort to confrontational strategies if necessary. Furthermore, unions with a one-dimensional market-orientated identity will gain more flexibility if they consider more confrontational strategies, especially if the preconditions for cooperative strategies repeatedly prove not to be met, as in the English cases. Unions have proven to be most successful where they could flexibly change between strategies or deploy several strategies simultaneously.

The high prerequisites of the partnership approach of formalization and complementing proactive strategies as part of a broader social agenda (Fichter and Greer 2004) should not be underestimated. As revealed in the corporatization and outsourcing case studies, this strategy requires high institutional power to secure trade union involvement, at least medium organizational and structural power to engage in complementary strategies and credibly threaten to resort to more confrontational action, as well as a certain degree of societal power to place the conflict in a broader social agenda. Organizing, social movement unionism, and lobbying necessitate other power resources. Organizing naturally requires high organizational power, but also a certain degree of structural power. To be able to successfully pursue a social movement unionism strategy, unions need to possess high societal power, as well as high organizational power. Last, but not least, a lobbying strategy can be an option if unions have access at the political level, societal power to exert public pressure if necessary, as well as a certain organizational power among affected workers to credibly speak on their behalf and exert pressure, as revealed in the staffing levels study from England. The power resource preconditions for each strategy are summarized in Table 7.2.

7.5 Contribution, shortcomings, and outlook

In this book, I presented 19 case studies in a structured, focused, and comparative design. The case studies were based on a broad empirical foundation and treated the three main forms of privatization – corporatization, outsourcing, and material privatization – as well as understaffing, one of their most severe effects. The studies were embedded in a most-different systems design, comparing liberal, and coordinated market economies, namely Germany and England, and, in the case of understaffing, the USA. With its design, the book focused on empirical evidence to contribute to the scarce literature on trade unionism in the health sector, especially in times of marketization and privatization.

In addition, the book developed a theoretical model that extends, refines and specifies the model of strategic union choice suggested by Frege and Kelly (2003), integrating different approaches to institutional change and employment relations, opportunity structures, and the trade union's local resources and capabilities, as well as the corresponding strategic choices. The theoretical part of this book aimed to review these approaches. The conclusion suggested their integration into a new coherent framework, suitable for studying trade union strategies in health sector marketization processes. It highlighted the strong effect of marketization processes in the hospital sector, superimposing national employment relations institutions. The theoretical framework emphasizes local-level variation, as well as the determining character of recognizing political opportunities stemming from marketization processes, local-level trade union resources and the unions' capability to deploy them. It also stresses the importance of capabilities and their interaction with power resources as a contribution to power resource theories. Ultimately, the theoretical model is intended to provide an analytical tool for trade union action and its prospects. It might facilitate the analysis of unions' scope for action, the detection of the weaknesses in and the potential of resources and capabilities, depending on which strategic choice can be made.

The book is of course not without shortcomings. After having presented the empirical material and the conclusions, it could be argued that the high number of case studies acted to the detriment of their depth. However, only by analyzing all main forms of marketization and its main effect of understaffing, could a holistic picture of trade unionism in times of hospital sector marketization be given. Furthermore, the comparison of the different conflict types emphasized how salience and societal power increase with the intensity of marketization.

Nevertheless, analyzing two different countries, four conflict types, and differing strategies yielded high complexity and much variation. The cases were nonetheless selected systematically. Their high variation in outcomes, or, in other words, strategic choices, supports the main argument of local-level variation, and the determining effect of local-level union resources and capabilities.

The generalization of the findings is limited as well. They might be transferable to other care sectors that experience increasing financial pressures and a high public interest in the services. Some of the findings might also be transferable to other sectors that are marked by low pay, high shares of women, and part-time employment. Chapter 6 has also shown that the theoretical framework developed for the comparison of England and Germany can also be used to study an understaffing-related conflict in New York State.

Further research is necessary to test the generalization of the findings. In this way, additional case studies in other care sectors or countries and a systematic Qualitative Comparative Analysis (QCA) (Rihoux and Ragin 2009) could help identify necessary and sufficient conditions for successful anti-marketization strategies in terms of salience, power resources, and capabilities. In addition, the case studies focused on the trade unions as organizations and were based at the meso-level. However, as is the case with any organization, there will be plurality and differing opinions about trade union action. Therefore, it would be interesting to complement the present studies with micro-level analyses. These could also target the question whether specific organizing and mobilization approaches are necessary for women, young workers, care workers, etc. Furthermore, these studies could take a closer look at challenges for local trade union officials to balance the interest of their union as a whole, and focus on their specific local-level leeways and conditions for strategic choices.

Last but not least, it should be reiterated that the analyses and implications for unions presented in this book take as given the structural conditions for the marketization of health care and the power imbalances between employees and employers. Ultimately, profound and sustainable change for better working conditions, adequate pay, high quality, and needs-based healthcare will require the attack of capitalist logics, driven by a broad social alliance.

References

Artus, Ingrid, Peter Birke, Stefan Kerber-Clasen, and Wolfgang Menz. 2017. *Sorge-Kämpfe: Auseinandersetzungen um Arbeit in sozialen Dienstleistungen.* Hamburg: VSA Verlag.

Baccaro, Lucio, Kerstin Hamann, and Lowell Turner. 2003. The Politics of Labour Movement Revitalization: The Need for a Revitalized Perspective. *European Journal of Industrial Relations* no. 9 (1):119–133.

Baccaro, Lucio, and Chris Howell. 2011. A Common Neoliberal Trajectory: The Transformation of Industrial Relations in Advanced Capitalism. *Politics & Society* no. 39 (4):521–563.

Behrens, Martin, Kerstin Hamann, and Richard Hurd. 2004. Conceptualizing Labor Union Revitalization. In *Varieties of Unionism: Strategies for Union Revitalization in a Globalizing Economy*, edited by Carola Frege and John Kelly, 11–30. Oxford/New York: Oxford University Press.

Bambra, Clare. 2005. Worlds of Welfare and the Health Care Discrepancy. *Social Policy and Society* no. 4 (1):31–41.

Benford, Robert D., and David A. Snow. 2000. Framing Processes and Social Movements: An Overview Assessment. *Annual Review of Sociology* no. 26 (1):611–639.

Bordogna, Lorenzo. 2008. Moral Hazard, Transaction Costs and the Reform of Public Service Employment Relations. *European Journal of Industrial Relations* no. 14 (4):381–400.

Briskin, Linda. 2012. Resistance, Mobilization and Militancy: Nurses on Strike. *Nursing Inquiry* no. 19 (4):285–296.

Chadwick, Ruth, and Alison Thompson. 2000. Professional Ethics and Labor Disputes: Medicine and Nursing in the United Kingdom. *Cambridge Quarterly of Healthcare Ethics* no. 9:483–497.

Culpepper, Pepper D. 2010. *Quiet Politics and Business Power: Corporate Control in Europe and Japan.* Cambridge, UK: Cambridge University Press.

Doellgast, Virginia, and Ian Greer. 2007. Vertical Disintegration and the Disorganization of German Industrial Relations. *British Journal of Industrial Relations* no. 45 (1):55–76.

Fichter, Michael, and Ian Greer. 2004. Analysing Social Partnership: A Tool of Union Revitalization?. In *Varieties of Unionism: Strategies for Union Revitalization in a Globalizing Economy*, edited by Carola Frege and John Kelly, 71–92. New York, NY: Oxford University Press.

Frege, Carola, Edmund Heery, and Lowell Turner. 2004. The New Solidarity? Trade Union Coalition-Building in Five Countries. In *Varieties of Unionism: Strategies for Union Revitalization in a Globalizing Economy*, edited by Carola Frege and John Kelly. Oxford/New York: Oxford University Press.

Frege, Carola, and John Kelly. 2003. Union Revitalization Strategies in Comparative Perspective. *European Journal of Industrial Relations* no. 9 (7):7–24.

Gamson, William A., and Davis S. Meyer. 1996. 12 - Framing Political Opportunity. In *Comparative Perspectives on Social Movements: Political Opportunities, Mobilizing Structures, and Cultural Framings*, edited by Dough McAdam, John D. McCarthy and Mayer N. Zald, 275–290.

Ganz, Marshall. 2000. Resources and Resourcefulness: Strategic Capacity in the Unionization of Californian Agriculture, 1959–1966. *The American Journal of Sociology* no. 105:1003–1062.

Ganz, Marshall. 2009. *Why David Sometimes Wins: Leadership, Organization, and Strategy in the California Farm Worker Movement*. Oxford/New York: Oxford University Press.

Gindin, Sam. 2016. Beyond Social Movement Unionism. *Jacobin*. https://www.jacobinmag.com/2016/08/beyond-social-movement-unionism/.

Hassel, Anke. 1999. The Erosion of the German System of Industrial Relations. *British Journal of Industrial Relations* no. 37 (3):483–505.

Hauptmeier, Marco. 2012. Institutions Are What Actors Make of Them — The Changing Construction of Firm-Level Employment Relations in Spain. *British Journal of Industrial Relations* no. 50 (4):737–759.

Hirschman, Albert O. 1970. *Exit, Voice, and Loyalty: Responses to Decline in Firms, Organizations, and States*. Cambridge, MA: Harvard University Press.

Hunt, Scott A., Robert D. Benford, and David A. Snow. 1994. Identity Fields: Framing Processes and the Social Construction of Movement Identities. In *New Social Movements: From Ideology to Identity*, edited by Enrique Laraña, Hank Johnston, Joseph R. Gusfield, 185–208. Philadelphia: Temple University Press.

Hyman, Richard. 2001. *Understanding European Trade Unionism*. London: SAGE.

Katz, Harry C., and Owen Darbishire. 2000. *Converging Divergences: Worldwide Changes in Employment Systems*. Ithaca/New York: ILR Press.

Kuypers, Jim A. 2009. Framing Analysis. In *Rhetorical Criticism: Perspectives in Action*, edited by Jim A. Kuypers, 181–204. Lanham and Plymouth: Lexington Books.

Lévesque, Christian, and Gregor Murray. 2010. Understanding Union Power: Resources and Capabilities for Renewing Union Capacity. *Transfer: European Review of Labour and Research* no. 16 (3):333–350.

Locke, Richard M. 1992. The Demise of the National Union in Italy: Lessons for Comparative Industrial Relations Theory. *Industrial & Labor Relations Review* no. 45 (2):229–249.

Nachtwey, Oliver, and Luigi Wolf. 2013. Strategisches Handlungsvermögen und Gewerkschaftliche Erneuerung im deutschen Modell industrieller Beziehungen. In *Comeback der Gewerkschaften? Machtressourcen, Innovative Praktiken, Internationale Perspektiven*, edited by Stefan Schmalz and Klaus Dörre, 104–123. Frankfurt am Main/New York: Campus.

Rihoux, Benoît, and Charles C. Ragin. 2009. *Configurational Comparative Methods: Qualitative Comparative Analysis (QCA) and Related Techniques, Applied Social Research Methods Series* Vol. 51. California: SAGE.

Streeck, Wolfgang, and Kathleen Thelen. 2005. *Beyond Continuity: Institutional Change in Advanced Political Economies.* New York, NY: Oxford University Press.

Tarrow, Sidney G.2011. *Power in Movement: Social Movements and Contentious Politics.* New York, NY: Cambridge University Press.

Turner, Lowell, and Richard W. Hurd. 2001. Building Social Movement Unionism. The Transformation of the American Labor Movement. In *Rekindling the Movement. Labor's Quest for Relevance in the 21st Century*, edited by Lowell Turner, Harry C. Katz and Richard W. Hurd, 9–26. Ithaca, NY: ILR Press.

Voss, Kim. 2010. Democratic Dilemmas: Union Democracy and Uinon Renewal. *Transfer* no. 16 (3): 369–382.

Wolf, Luigi. 2015. Mehr von uns ist besser für alle: die Streiks an der Berliner Charité und ihre Bedeutung für die Aufwertung von Care-Arbeit. In *UMCARE: Gesundheit und Pflege neu organisieren*, edited by Barbara Fried and Hannah Schurian, 23–31. Berlin: Rosa-Luxemburg-Stiftung.

Index

For Product Safety Concerns and Information please contact our EU
representative GPSR@taylorandfrancis.com
Taylor & Francis Verlag GmbH, Kaufingerstraße 24, 80331 München, Germany